Lecture Notes on
Clinical Investigation

D1627745

Lecture Notes on Clinical Investigation

EDITED BY
DEREK MACLEAN
PhD, FRCP, FRCP(E)
Unit Medical Manager,
Dundee General Hospital

MALCOLM BATESON
MD, FRCP, FRCP(E)
Consultant Physician,
Bishop Auckland General Hospital

CHRISTOPHER PENNINGTON
MD, BSc, FRCP(E)
Consultant Physician,
University of Dundee

OXFORD

BLACKWELL SCIENTIFIC PUBLICATIONS

LONDON EDINBURGH BOSTON

MELBOURNE PARIS BERLIN VIENNA

© 1991 by
Blackwell Scientific Publications
Editorial Offices:
Osney Mead, Oxford OX2 0EL
25 John Street, London WC1N 2BL
23 Ainslie Place, Edinburgh EH3 6AJ
3 Cambridge Center, Cambridge
    Massachusetts 02142, USA
54 University Street, Carlton
    Victoria 3053, Australia

Other Editorial Offices:
Arnette SA
2, rue Casimir-Delavigne
75006 Paris
France

Blackwell Wissenschaft
Meinekestrasse 4
D-1000 Berlin 15
Germany

Blackwell MZV
Feldgasse 13
A-1238 Wien
Austria

First published 1991

Set by Semantic Graphics, Singapore
Printed and bound in Great Britain by
Hartnolls Ltd, Bodmin, Cornwall

DISTRIBUTORS

Marston Book Services Ltd
PO Box 87
Oxford OX2 0DT
(*Orders*: Tel. 0865 791155
       Fax: 0865 791927
       Telex: 837515)

USA
Mosby-Year Book, Inc.
11830 Westline Industrial Drive
St Louis, Missouri 63146
(*Orders*: Tel: (800) 663-6699)

Canada
Mosby-Year Book, Inc.
5240 Finch Avenue East
Scarborough, Ontario
(*Orders*: Tel: (416) 298-1588)

Australia
Blackwell Scientific Publications
(Australia) Pty Ltd
54 University Street
Carlton, Victoria 3053
(*Orders*: Tel: (03) 347-0300)

British Library
Cataloguing in Publication Data

Lecture notes on Clinical Investigation.
    1. Medicine. Diagnosis. Tests. Assessment
    I. Maclean, Derek   II. Bateson,
    Malcolm C. (Malcolm Cedric), *1945–*
    III. Pennington, Christopher Royston
    616.075

ISBN 0-632-02907-2

Contents

List of Contributors

C.B. BALLINGER MRCP, FRCPsych,
Consultant Psychiatrist, Dundee Mental Health Unit; Hon. Senior Lecturer, Department of Psychiatry, University of Dundee

M.C. BATESON MD, FRCP, FRCP(E),
Consultant Gastrointestinal Physician, Bishop Auckland General Hospital

G.R.D. CATTO MD, DSc, FRCP, FRCP(E), FRCP(G),
Professor of Medicine and Therapeutics, University of Aberdeen; Hon. Consultant Physician/Nephrologist, Grampian Health Board

H.W. CLAGUE BSc, MD, MRCP,
Consultant Physician and Specialist in Respiratory Medicine, Bishop Auckland General Hospital

R.S. CLARK MRCP,
Consultant Cardiological Physician, Scarborough Hospital, Scarborough

D.L.W. DAVIDSON BSc, FRCP(E),
Consultant Neurologist, Dundee Royal Infirmary; Hon. Senior Lecturer in Medicine, University of Dundee

A.J. McCULLOCH BSc, MD, FRCP, FRCP(E),
Consultant Physician, Bishop Auckland General Hospital

K.D. MORLEY FRCP(E), FRACP,
Consultant Physician, Ninewells Hospital, Dundee; Hon. Senior Lecturer in Medicine, University of Dundee

S.M. MORLEY MD, MRCP, FRACP,
Senior Registrar in Dermatology, Ninewells Hospital, Dundee

A.J. NICHOLLS MRCP,
Consultant Physician/Nephrologist, Royal Devon and Exeter Hospital (Wonford)

N.B. PATEL FRCOG,
Consultant Obstetrician, Ninewells Hospital, Dundee; Hon. Senior Lecturer in Obstetrics, University of Dundee

C.R. PENNINGTON BSc, MD, FRCP(E),
Consultant Physician (Gastroenterology), Ninewells Hospital, Dundee; Hon. Senior Lecturer in Clinical Pharmacology, University of Dundee

P.E. PREECE   MD(Wales), FRCS(E), FRCS(Eng),
Senior Lecturer in Surgery, University of Dundee; Hon. Consultant Surgeon, Ninewells Hospital, Dundee

J.S. SCOTT   FRCR, FFR, DMRT,
Consultant Radiotherapist and Oncological Physician, Ninewells Hospital, Dundee; Director: Tayside Area Radiotherapy and Oncology Service; Hon. Senior Lecturer in Radiotherapy and Oncology, University of Dundee (Retired)

R A SHARP   MRCP, MRCPath
Senior Registrar in Haematology, Ninewells Hospital, Dundee; Hon. Lecturer in Haematology, University of Dundee

G.R. TUDHOPE   MD, BSc, FRCP, FRCP(E),
Reader in Therapeutics, Department of Pharmacology and Clinical Pharmacology, University of Dundee; Hon. Consultant Physician, Ninewells Hospital, Dundee (Retired)

E.M. WALKER   MD, MRCOG,
Lecturer, Department of Obstetrics and Gynaecology, Ayrshire Central Hospital, Irvine

M.G. WALKER   ChM, FRCS,
Consultant Vascular Surgeon, Manchester Royal Infirmary

Preface

This book is designed as an aid to planning investigations needed after the patient has been questioned and physically examined. A large panel of authors actively practising clinical medicine has been recruited to give a discerning up-to-date assessment of the place of different tests used in confirming or refuting diagnoses. Emphasis is placed on those tests of greatest practical use and on tests which should normally be freely available either in District General Hospitals or, where appropriate, in centres of specialist referral. The chapters are organized by major systems since it should generally be clear which organs are apparently malfunctioning. The book is designed for medical students and postgraduate students preparing for higher examinations, but it should also be a useful rapid reference text for the clinician practising internal medicine.

J.S. Scott contributed to several sections on aspects of oncology and radiotherapy.

D.M.
M.C.B.
C.R.P.

Introduction

The onset of disease, other than trivial ailments, has important implications for patients and their medical attendants. Many disorders cannot be diagnosed with confidence by clinical methods alone, and clinical examination frequently provides little information about the severity or cause of the illness in the individual patient. Clinical investigation is thus required to establish a diagnosis, identify the cause of the disease, define its severity, and monitor the response to treatment.

The rapid progress in our understanding of disease, which has led to major improvements in treatment, has been accompanied by corresponding advances in investigative techniques. The introduction of imaging by computerized (axial) tomography, nuclear magnetic resonance and ultrasound, and the development of fibreoptic instruments represent examples of important improvements in the methods of patient management. These in turn have further enhanced our understanding of the diseases under investigation.

The increasing number and spectrum of investigative techniques calls for careful selection for safe and cost-effective practice. New methods should replace older techniques where there is a demonstrable improvement in the accuracy of the information and patient safety. The tendency to use new methods as an adjunct to traditional investigations should be resisted unless they are complementary. Furthermore, there should always be a clear idea of the purpose of each investigation. The nature of the information which may be gleaned has to be set against any risk to the patient and the financial cost.

This book reviews the methods of investigation which are currently used in clinical practice. Chapters are set out under organ systems. A review of the clinical features of the disorders affecting each system is followed by a description of individual investigations and a summary in which the method of investigation and the use of various techniques is outlined.

Chapter 1
Gastroenterology

Introduction

The history is crucial in planning the approach to diagnosis but physical examination is often disappointingly unhelpful, so that targeted investigations are of prime importance.

Common problems for evaluation are given in Table 1.1. Such symptoms may reflect pathology in specific parts of the gastrointestinal tract, liver or pancreas, and the use of techniques for their investigation is the subject of this chapter. However, it must be remembered that the majority of these features can occur for reasons other than gastrointestinal disease. Thus, anorexia, vomiting and diarrhoea may be caused by drug toxicity or renal failure, and jaundice may be due to congestive cardiac failure or haemolysis.

The next section briefly summarizes common symptoms and the subsequent two sections review investigative techniques and their application.

General symptoms

The problems which patients present for investigation are given in Table 1.1. Terms such as flatulence and dyspepsia have not been included; the former as a single symptom rarely signifies disease and the latter lacks specificity. Furthermore, many patients regard diarrhoea as stool frequency, but this term should be applied to watery or loose stool.

Heartburn is a very common symptom caused by gastro-oesophageal reflux leading to inflammation of the oesophageal mucosa; if severe, fibrosis and stricturing ensues causing dysphagia. Dysphagia also results from oesophageal carcinoma. Pain in the chest, which can mimic coronary artery insufficiency, is frequently due to oesophageal dysmotility. Oesophageal spasm may reflect reflux oesophagitis or a primary motility disorder.

A variety of disorders from depression to malignancy lead to anorexia; in older patients it may be due to gastric carcinoma. Upper abdominal pain is caused by disease of the stomach and duodenum, gallbladder or pancreas. Peptic ulcer pain is often described as burning in nature and is not usually severe; night-waking and relief from food are common features. Pain from cholelithiasis

Table 1.1 Common problems in gastroenterology

Heartburn	Constipation
Chest pain	Gastrointestinal bleeding
Dysphagia	Anaemia
Anorexia	Jaundice
Abdominal pain	Malabsorption and weight loss
Vomiting	Ascites
Diarrhoea	

is colicky and may radiate from the epigastrium to the back; that of pancreatic origin is often felt as a prolonged deep boring pain which radiates through to the back. Mid-abdominal pain may be caused by disease of the small intestine, and pain in the lower abdomen arises from the colon as well as the pelvic organs.

Vomiting may be due to gastroduodenal disease, pyloric or intestinal obstruction (when it is copious) as well as infection, drug therapy, and raised intracranial pressure. There are several mechanisms of diarrhoea. Secretory diarrhoea leads to the production of watery stool; it occurs with infections such as cholera and salmonella as well as with rare endocrine-secreting tumours. Malabsorptive diarrhoea leads to the passage of pale, offensive stool which contains an excessive amount of fat; it is associated with small bowel and pancreatic disease. Colloid diarrhoea is a result of exudation across inflamed intestinal mucosa when the stool contains blood, as in inflammatory bowel disease and certain forms of intestinal infection.

Constipation occurs with colonic disease, particularly carcinoma, when a change in bowel habit is important. On the other hand, it may simply reflect immobility and poor diet in the elderly patient, concomitant drug therapy, or hypercalcaemia. Jaundice can signify haemolysis, liver disease, or biliary obstruction.

The patient who presents with anaemia often requires gastrointestinal investigation for malabsorption or blood loss. Blood loss is dramatic and obvious with bleeding ulcers or oesophageal varices; the patient vomits fresh or altered blood (coffee grounds) or passes partly digested blood per rectum (melaena stool).

Individual investigations will be discussed first. They are summarized in Table 1.2, and then their application to specific symptoms will be reviewed.

Specific investigations

The investigations commonly employed are summarized in Table 1.2.

Endoscopy

The introduction of flexible fibreoptic endoscopes has revolutionized the practice of gastroenterology. Each endoscope conforms to a basic design. The fibreoptic light bundle transmits the light and the image; there are channels to blow air and water, to apply suction and to allow the passage of biopsy forceps, catheters and cytology brushes. The flexible tip is guided by wires which pass down the instrument and are controlled by wheels so that a wide range of view may be obtained. This system is currently being replaced by video endoscopy which involves the use of distal light sensors with electrical transmission of images to television screens. There are a variety of instrument widths and lengths designed

Table 1.2 Common investigative techniques in gastroenterology

Endoscopy	Blood tests
Radiography	Stool examination
Nuclear medicine	Manometry
Histopathology	

for paediatric or adult practice, gastroscopy or colonoscopy. All the instruments must be maintained with care; meticulous cleaning is vital to prevent the transmission of infection including hepatitis B and the HIV agent.

Upper alimentary endoscopy

Upper alimentary endoscopy is indicated for the investigation of oesophageal and gastroduodenal symptoms. It may identify oesophageal disease such as peptic oesophagitis, strictures and carcinomas, gastric and duodenal ulcers and carcinoma of the stomach. Endoscopy is essential to diagnose a bleeding source. It may also be required for the dilatation of oesophageal strictures and the injection of oseophageal varices. A more recent indication involves the use of laser treatment for the palliation of oesophageal carcinoma and the arrest of bleeding ulcers (the latter may be achieved more easily with a heat probe passed down the endoscope). Contra-indications include a haemodynamically unstable patient and cardiorespiratory failure so that the patient cannot lie supine.

The patient must be fasting and after any dentures are removed most prefer to receive intravenous sedation with diazepam emulsion or midazolam to achieve drowsiness and amnesia; some endoscopists also use a topical anaesthetic throat spray and an anti-cholinergic to reduce motility. The instrument is passed through a protective mouth guard with the patient in the left lateral position and advanced into the oesophagus as the patient swallows, and ultimately into the duodenum with careful inspection.

Complications are rare. They include complications of oversedation, gastric aspiration and trauma. A careless insertion can rupture the oesophagus.

Endoscopic retrograde cholangio-pancreatography (ERCP)

In this technique a side-viewing endoscope is used and positioned with the end adjacent to the ampulla of Vater. A cannula is passed through the biopsy channel and into the ampulla, radiographic contrast is injected to outline the biliary tree and pancreas.

ERCP has a diagnostic role in patients with chronic pancreatitis or carcinoma, sclerosing cholangitis and retained bile duct stones, as well as a therapeutic role in the retrieval of retained bile duct stones and stent insertion for strictures. The former requires the enlargement of the exit from the bile duct by sphincterotomy; this involves the passage of a bowed catheter with a wire which is used to cut the ampullary orifice with an electric current.

It is a difficult procedure which is not universally available. Complications include pancreatitis and cholangitis. Sphincterotomy may cause haemorrhage which can require surgical intervention. It should be performed with antibiotic prophylaxis.

Flexible sigmoidoscopy

The 60 cm flexible sigmoidoscope offers excellent visualization of the distal colon and rectum, often as far as the splenic flexure. A phosphate enema readily clears the left side of the bowel. The procedure is performed in the left lateral position without sedation. This is the first investigation for the evaluation of rectal bleeding. Other indications include the investigation of a change in bowel habit and the delineation of the extent of distal colitis.

Colonoscopy

Instruments up to 180 cm long permit the inspection of the remainder of the colon in most, but not all, patients. Adequate bowel preparation with an osmotic laxative is essential. The procedure can be very time-consuming and sedation is required.

Indications for colonoscopy include the diagnosis of inflammatory bowel disease, the diagnosis and removal (by diathermy snare which is passed down the biopsy channel) of polyps, the investigation of colonic bleeding and the pursuit of equivocal radiological findings. It will allow the diagnosis of polyps, carcinomas, inflammatory bowel disease and angiodysplasia.

Serious complications include perforation and bleeding. Perforation is more likely with excessive sedation and distended bowel loops; bleeding can follow polypectomy.

Laparoscopy

Laparoscopy has long been used by gynaecologists; its application in gastro-intestinal practice is more recent and much less frequent. The abdomen is distended with gas (CO_2 or N_2), usually with the patient under general anaesthesia, and the laparoscope is inserted through the abdominal wall. The internal organs are inspected and target biopsies obtained. Laparoscopy is used for the investigation of abdominal pain as well as the investigation and staging of malignancy. It is difficult or impossible after surgery because of adhesions; under these circumstances complications such as damage to the intestine are more likely.

Radiography, ultrasonography and magnetic resonance

This is a rapidly changing field in which there are developments of both diagnostic and therapeutic techniques. Methods of radiographic diagnoses are summarized in Table 1.3. Care must be taken to minimize exposure to radiation; methods using X-rays must not be used during pregnancy unless unavoidable.

Table 1.3 Gastrointestinal imaging techniques

Imaging techniques
    Ultrasound
    Computerized tomography
    Nuclear magnetic resonance

Barium examinations
    Barium meal
    Small bowel enema
    Barium enema

Miscellaneous
    Plain abdominal film
    Oral cholecystogram
    Intravenous cholangiogram
    Percutaneous cholangiogram
    Fistulogram

The plain abdominal X-ray

This may provide evidence of intestinal obstruction and will sometimes suggest the level at which the bowel is obstructed. It is an important tool in the management of acute colitis when it may show dilatation of the colon, or proximal faecal loading with distal disease. A perforated viscus is suggested by gas under the diaphragm. Calcification may be seen in chronic pancreatitis and a minority of gallstones.

Ultrasound

This is a most useful non-invasive method which is commonly employed to examine the liver and biliary tree. It is the method of choice for seeking gallstones, hepatic metastases and pancreatic tumours. The presence, and sometimes the cause, of biliary obstruction may be determined in the jaundiced patient. Ultrasound guidance is useful for target biopsies and the percutaneous drainage of hepatic abscesses.

Computerized tomography

This is also used to explore mass lesions in the liver, pancreas or retroperitoneal regions, particularly when poor acoustic access has prevented visualization by ultrasound. As with ultrasound, it is useful for guided biopsy.

Barium studies

Barium meal

Even though modern double-contrast examinations are almost as accurate as endoscopy for the demonstration of ulcers, it is less useful in the detection of oesophagitis and early gastric cancer; therefore direct inspection by endoscopy with target biopsy is the preferred investigation for upper alimentary symptoms. Exceptions include the investigation of suspected oesophageal motility disorders. Radiography is also required in patients who are unfit for endoscopy.

Small bowel examination

This is performed either by asking the patient to swallow barium and following its passage down the intestine, or by running the barium through a tube directly into the duodenum. The latter method gives better results. These studies are used to identify Crohn's disease or small intestinal lymphomas.

Barium enema

This is a technique which is regarded with considerable trepidation by patients, sometimes not without reason! The obligatory bowel preparation is the least popular part of the exercise; air insufflation to produce double-contrast pictures may also cause discomfort. Barium enemas are used to look for inflammatory bowel disease, polyps and carcinomas. Diverticular disease will be clearly demonstrated. In most centres it is used before consideration of the more time-consuming colonoscopy, although sigmoidoscopy should precede a barium examination as the latter may miss lesions in the rectum and distal sigmoid colon.

Fistulogram
Internal fistulae between loops of bowel will usually be identified on a barium enema or small bowel study. A fistulogram is often helpful to locate the source of an enterocutaneous fistula.

Radiography of the biliary tract
Many of the older techniques have been superseded.

Oral cholecystography
This involves the ingestion of a radiopaque dye that is absorbed, taken up by the liver and subsequently concentrated in the gallbladder. Gallstones are thus outlined as filling defects. Failure to opacify is taken as evidence of a non-functioning gallbladder with a blocked cystic duct; it might also be due to the failure to absorb the contrast medium. Ultrasound is the preferred investigation for gallstones; however, an oral cholecystogram may still be useful in assessing the suitability of stones for dissolution therapy when a functioning gallbladder is required.

Intravenous cholangiography
This involves the intravenous infusion of contrast media to opacify the biliary tree including the gallbladder. Unfortunately, this method fails in the presence of jaundice, the very situation when it would be most valuable. Adverse reactions to the contrast media and impairment of renal function are other disadvantages of the method which has now been replaced by ultrasound and ERCP in most centres.

Percutaneous trans-hepatic cholangiogram
A fine needle is inserted into the liver substance and contrast injected under screening as it is slowly withdrawn in the hope of opacifying the biliary tree via the intrahepatic radicles. Whereas it has largely been superseded by ERCP, it is still used to identify the upper limit of a stricture, when ERCP fails, and as a preliminary to the stenting of a high stricture. Coagulation defects and ascites are contra-indications; bleeding and infection are potential complications.

Vascular studies
Angiography is required occasionally to identify the source of obscure intestinal bleeding or to delineate the vascular supply to a tumour before embolization.

Nuclear medicine

Hepatic and biliary imaging
Compounds have been developed which are rapidly excreted by the liver even in the presence of jaundice. Iminodiacetic compounds (HIDA) are most widely used. In normal individuals intravenous administration leads to a rapid accumulation in the gallbladder. In acute cholecystitis there is activity in the liver and bile

ducts but not in the gallbladder. In the jaundiced patient delayed excretion may suggest biliary obstruction. The faecal excretion of radioactivity in children can be used to differentiate biliary atresia where excretion is normal, and neonatal hepatitis where it is low.

Technetium isotopes have been used to obtain an image of the liver, particularly for the investigation of metastatic disease when tumour masses which do not take up the isotope cause many filling defects. Hepatoma cells sometimes take up selenium; this led to the use of technetium followed by selenium in such patients. However, these methods have been replaced by newer methods of imaging.

Nuclear medicine in the assessment of motility

Radionuclide studies may be used to investigate oesophageal dysmotility. The patient drinks a small amount of technetium-99m (^{99m}Tc) colloid while lying under a scintiscanner; radioactivity is normally cleared from the oesophagus within 15 s. Oesophageal dysmotility is shown by persistence of radioactivity in the oesophagus. It may oscillate backwards and forwards as in diffuse oesophageal spasm, or remain static as in achlasia. Gastro-oesophageal reflux may be shown, either spontaneous or after applied extra-abdominal pressure.

Gastric emptying may be determined for both liquid and solid phase by giving the patient appropriately labelled drinks such as orange juice and dextrin mixed with technetium or meals such as scrambled eggs labelled with technetium.

Tests of digestive and absorptive function

Glycocholate breath test

This is used to investigate small bowel bacterial overgrowth which impairs digestive function. It is based on the ability of most intestinal bacteria to deconjugate bile acids. This normally only occurs to any significant extent in the colon. If there is colonization of the upper small bowel, deconjugation of [^{14}C]glycine–glycocholic acid liberates ^{14}C-labelled glycine which is metabolized to $^{14}CO_2$. This can then be measured in the breath. Obviously the test is influenced by changes in intestinal transit and biliary infection.

Triolein breath test

This can be used to investigate pancreatic function. A tracer dose of the triglyceride glyceryl-[^{14}C]triolein is given with a standard carrier meal of known fat content. Each of the three oleic acid molecules in the triglyceride is labelled with carbon-14, and after digestion they are absorbed and metabolized to $^{14}CO_2$ and H_2O, the $^{14}CO_2$ is exhaled and the amount of radioactive $^{14}CO_2$ relates to the digestion of the triglyceride. Over 6 h normal subjects excrete more than 9% of the administered dose; in steatorrhoea excretion is less than 6%. Misleading results may be obtained in patients with respiratory disease or obesity. An abnormal result will also be obtained in patients who have absorptive impairment (gluten enteropathy) as well as digestive impairment (pancreatic exocrine insufficiency).

Schilling test

This measures the absorption of vitamin B_{12}. The body stores of this vitamin are first saturated with an intramuscular injection so that any of the labelled vitamin which is subsequently given by mouth and absorbed will be excreted in the urine. In a normal person more than 10% of the oral dose is detected in the urine. Clearly, impaired absorption may reflect a deficiency of intrinsic factor (pernicious anaemia or gastrectomy), bacterial overgrowth or disease of the terminal ileum. Using a double isotope, ^{57}Co-cobalamin bound to intrinsic factor, and free ^{58}Co-cobalamin, it is possible to determine if intrinsic factor deficiency is present by examining the ratio of excreted isotopes. This test is dependent on accurate urine collections and good renal function.

Miscellaneous applications

Inflammatory response attracts leucocytes. Labelling the patient's own leucocytes *in vitro* with indium or technetium followed by re-injection, will permit the localization of infection or abscesses by scanning with a gamma camera. The same approach has been used to assess the extent and localization of inflammatory bowel disease. Such methods lack sensitivity and specificity; they are not universally accepted.

Re-injection of red cells labelled with ^{99m}Tc has been used to find the source of obscure intestinal bleeding. Furthermore, the abnormal location of hydrogen ion secretion in patients with Meckel's diverticulum can be identified by the intravenous injection of ^{99m}Tc as pertechnecate.

Protein-losing enteropathy can be identified by an intravenous injection of chromium-51 chloride as a method for the *in vivo* labelling of serum protein. Stools are collected for 5 days, during which time normal subjects excrete less than 1% of the injected radioactivity.

Histopathology

Histopathology plays a very important role in gastroenterology. Biopsy specimens may be obtained via the endoscope, at operation, or by percutaneous biopsy of organs such as the liver.

The pathologist is required to identify the nature of the pathology and sometimes to comment on the response to treatment. For example, changes in the liver histology which accompany the institution of steroid treatment in chronic active hepatitis, or the recovery of the villi following the introduction of a gluten-free diet in patients with gluten enteropathy.

The role of histopathology is summarized in Table 1.4.

Percutaneous liver biopsies are indicated for the investigation of suspected chronic liver disease, such as chronic persistent hepatitis, chronic active hepatitis and primary biliary cirrhosis. It is sometimes required in the investigation of alcohol-or drug-induced liver injury, iron or copper storage disease, malignancy and various rare disorders. Such biopsies should not be attempted in the presence of extrahepatic cholestasis, gross ascites, or significant coagulation defect (platelet count less than $100 \times 10^9 \, 1^{-1}$ or prothrombin time more than 3 s prolonged). Samples are obtained from the supine patient in the right lateral position over the point of maximum liver dullness. Either suction Menghini or

Table 1.4 The role of pathological investigation

Organ	Specimen	Disease
Oesophagus	Endoscopic biopsy Surgical resection	Oesophagitis Barrett's epithelium Carcinoma Candidiasis CMV infection
Stomach	Endoscopic biopsy Surgical resection	Gastritis *Helicobacter* infection Gastric ulcer Carcinoma Lymphoma
Small bowel	Endoscopic biopsy (distal duodenal) Crosby capsule Surgical resection	Gluten enteropathy Crohn's disease Giardiasis Lymphoma Carcinoma Whipple's disease
Colon and rectum	Endoscopic biopsy Surgical resection	Carcinoma Ulcerative colitis Crohn's disease Pseudomembraneous colitis Polyps Melanosis coli Amyloidosis
Liver	Percutaneous biopsy Surgical resection	Chronic persistent hepatitis Chronic active hepatitis Alcoholic liver disease Primary biliary cirrhosis Glycogen storage disease Amyloidosis Tuberculosis Carcinoma
Pancreas	Fine needle aspiration Operative resection	Chronic pancreatitis Carcinoma

disposable TruCut needles may be used to yield equivalent results. Significant complications can occur. They include the perforation of an adjacent viscus, such as the gallbladder or hepatic flexure of the colon, and haemorrhage. This investigation should not be performed without good indication.

The Crosby–Kugler capsule consists of a small capsule which contains a rotation spring-activated knife and which is attached to a metre of narrow tubing. The knife is loaded and the fasting patient swallows the capsule and part of the tubing. When the capsule reaches the proximal jejunum, suction is applied to the end of the tubing which draws a sample of mucosa into a window and at the same time activates the knife, thereby slicing this specimen of mucosa which is retrieved as the capsule is withdrawn. These specimens are usually obtained to investigate the possibility of gluten enteropathy, or to assess the response to dietary treatment. Complications are very uncommon.

Blood tests

Biochemistry

Liver function tests
The tests which are commonly regarded as liver function tests are summarized in Table 1.5.

It is apparent that all these tests lack specificity; many also lack sensitivity. The only true liver function test is the prothrombin time; persistent prolongation after vitamin K replacement reflects significant liver impairment. Albumin is another protein synthesized in the liver; however, reduced values are found with fluid shifts and malnutrition as well as in hepatic disease.

Table 1.5 Liver function tests

Measurement	Conditions in which increased values occur
Bilirubin	Haemolysis, liver disease and biliary obstruction
Alkaline phosphatase	Biliary tract disease, intrahepatic cholestasis, hepatic space-occupying lesions, bone disease—osteomalacia, intestinal disease
Transaminases	Hepatitis, hepatic necrosis Muscle disease—myositis Myocardial infarction
Gamma-glutamyl transpeptidase	As for alkaline phosphatase, but readily induced—drugs, ethanol
Prothrombin time	Hepatic disease-impaired synthesis, cholestasis—vitamin K deficiency

Interpretation of the pattern of abnormalities is sometimes helpful. Very high transaminase values occur early in the course of viral hepatitis or with paracetamol overdose; however, patients may subsequently enter a cholestatic phase on recovering from hepatitis with a predominant elevation of the alkaline phosphatase level. High bilirubin and alkaline phosphatase values imply cholestasis and the urgent need to seek or exclude biliary obstruction. Very high alkaline phosphatase values occur with metastatic disease when the bilirubin value is often normal and in primary biliary cirrhosis. The disproportionate increase in gamma-glutamyl transpeptidase in comparison with alkaline phosphatase suggests drug induction and particularly ethanol abuse. These abnormalities are summarized in Table 1.6.

Amylase
Amylase is released from the pancreas during acute pancreatitis, grossly elevated serum values (fivefold elevation or at least 1000 iu ml^{-1}) support this diagnosis. There are other sources of serum amylase, including the parotid glands.

Table 1.6 Pattern of biochemical abnormalities in hepatobiliary disease

	VH	AH	BOB	SOL
B	2	3	4	0–1
AP	1	2	3	4
AST	4	2	2	0–1
GGTP	1	4	3	3

Abbreviations: B = bilirubin; AP = alkaline phosphatase; AST = aspartate aminotransferase; GGTP = gamma-glutamyl transpeptidase; VH = viral hepatitis; AH = alcoholic hepatitis; BOB = bile duct obstruction; SOL = space-occupying lesion. 1–4 represents a range of relative increase which will vary according to the stage and severity of the disease.

Electrolytes

Patients with diarrhoea lose electrolytes in the stool. Those who abuse laxatives in particular are prone to hypokalaemia, mainly due to renal loss through secondary hyperaldosteronism which accompanies chronic saline depletion. Patients with Crohn's disease, particularly involving the small intestine, develop magnesium depletion. Very low serum zinc is found in patients with acrodermatitis enteropathica.

Vitamin D

Patients with fat malabsorption, including gluten enteropathy, pancreatic exocrine insufficiency, primary biliary cirrhosis and the short-bowel syndrome, may develop osteomalacia. They will have low serum calcium values (after correction for hypo-albuminaemia) and elevated serum alkaline phosphatase values. The metabolite 25-hydroxy vitamin D can be measured as a guide to the vitamin D status.

Miscellaneous biochemical tests

The serum iron is usually elevated in disorders of overload. In haemochromatosis the transferrin is 80–100% saturated compared with the normal 30–40% saturation. Low serum iron values occur in iron deficiency and inflammatory disorders such as rheumatoid arthritis. The transferrin is elevated in iron deficiency but not with inflammatory diseases. Low transferrin concentrations occur in malnutrition.

Copper-carrying caeruloplasmin levels are low in Wilson's disease when urinary copper excretion is enhanced.

Haematology

A full blood count provides important information. A microcytic hypochromic anaemia is suggestive of iron deficiency; this can be confirmed by measuring the iron and transferrin levels (see above). Apart from menorrhagia and a poor diet (an uncommon cause of deficiency in the UK except in the context of disease-associated anorexia), such a finding prompts consideration of poor absorption or blood loss.

A macrocytic blood film, in the absence of haemolysis, suggests the possibility of ethanol abuse which is sometimes accompanied by a sideroblastic anaemia or thrombocytopenia. A macrocytic anaemia particularly suggests the need to consider folate deficiency, dietary or malabsorptive, or vitamin B_{12} deficiency. The latter may follow gastrectomy, atrophic gastritis, or ileal resection.

Folate and vitamin B_{12} can be measured in serum samples to confirm these suspicions. The ability to absorb vitamin B_{12} is measured by the Schilling test which has been described previously.

Viral tests

Serological tests for viral infections are important. Those most commonly requested are for hepatitis viruses. Hepatitis A is very common in the community as a cause of clinical or subclinical acute hepatitis, but not of chronic liver disease. Because of its prevalence the finding of IgG antibodies to the hepatitis A virus provides little information about the cause of jaundice in a given patient. In this context IgM antibodies should be requested; they remain elevated for about 6 weeks.

The serological response to hepatitis B is summarized in Fig. 1.1. This virus is usually recognized by the detection of the surface antigen, HB_sAg. During an acute infection in which the virus is usually cleared, the surface antigen may disappear before the surface antibody (anti-HB_s) can be measured. Thus, the core antibody (anti-HB_c) is also sought. It is probably the most sensitive index of previous or present infection. The third antigen system is the e antigen, HB_eAg. The presence of this antigen correlates with the viral DNA polymerase activity and implies high infectivity. Patients become less infectious as they seroconvert to clear the e antigen when e antibodies (anti-HB_e) can be found. Because many of the 10% of patients who fail to clear the B virus develop chronic liver disease and/or hepatoma, viral markers should be sought in those circumstances.

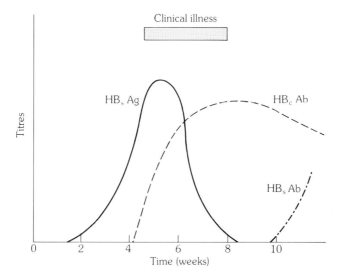

Fig. 1.1 Serological responses to hepatitis B infection. Abbreviations: HB_sAg = surface antigen; HB_sAb = surface antibody; HB_cAb = core antibody.

Finally, the D (Delta) virus is an incomplete RNA agent which infects only those patients who harbour the B virus and leads to severe acute and chronic hepatitis. Antibodies should be sought in drug addicts who are at particular risk of delta hepatitis.

Other forms of viral hepatitis exist including the recently identified C virus. Serology (anti-HCV) for this agent is appropriate in otherwise unexplained acute hepatitis and chronic liver disease, particularly because effective therapy is now available in the form of interferon.

Screening for the HIV agents should be considered in those at risk with diarrhoea and weight loss. In patients with this infection other viral diseases may be present but these usually require confirmation by histology or other means.

Miscellaneous blood tests

The mitochondrial antibody is present in 90% of patients with primary biliary cirrhosis. Smooth muscle antibody and antinuclear factor are found in many patients with lupoid-type chronic active hepatitis.

Serum gastrin values are very high in patients with gastrinomas (Zollinger–Ellison syndrome) and the excluded antrum syndrome. Similarly, a vipoma which presents with watery diarrhoea and hypokalaemia can be detected by measuring the vasoactive intestinal peptide.

Alpha-fetoprotein can usually be detected in the serum of patients with hepatoma, as well as in women carrying fetuses with spinal malformations. Carcino-embryonic and oncofetal antigens are markers of colonic and pancreatic carcinomas respectively. They are unreliable in diagnosis, but they may be useful in monitoring progress in established disease to detect tumour recurrence or response to treatment.

Tests of stool

Much can be learned from simple stool inspection. Blood and mucus suggest colonic inflammation, pale porridgy stool implies malabsorption, black tarry stool is indicative of upper gastrointestinal bleeding. Fluid stool in the absence of food intake is suggestive of a secretory diarrhoea, most commonly due to bacterial infection. A stool weight under 250 g per day implies that the patient is not suffering from diarrhoea, even though he may have stool frequency due to a motility disorder.

Faecal blood tests

The normal person loses about 0.7 ml of blood in the stool each day, a daily loss of more than 100 ml is required to produce melaena; between these extremes special tests are required to identify bleeding from the intestinal tract.

Chemical tests for faecal occult blood are based on the peroxidase-like activity on iron in haemoglobin which causes reagents to develop a blue colour; examples include Hema–Chek and the Feca–Twin tests. These tests all involve a compromise between false positive results in response to physiological bleeding or dietary ingredients and false negative results due to lack of sensitivity. Furthermore, it must be remembered that many tumours bleed intermittently.

Faecal fat excretion

The patient is given a standard 100 g fat diet and the stools are collected over 3 or 5 days. Normal subjects excrete less than 17 mmol of fat per day in the stool. Moderately elevated values are found in conditions which cause malabsorption, such as gluten enteropathy, giardiasis and bacterial overgrowth. Severe steatorrhoea occurs with pancreatic exocrine failure when the patient may excrete more than five times the normal amount of fat. This test is unpopular for obvious reasons with both patient and laboratory. A single normal value in a patient in whom malabsorption is reasonably suspected should not be assumed to exclude it.

Microbiology of the stool

Patients suspected of intestinal infections should have their stool examined by microscopy and culture. The former may identify protozoa such as *Giardia lamblia*, *Entamoeba histolytica* and cryptococci, as well as worm infestations. The latter seeks bacterial pathogens such as *Campylobacter jejuni*, *Salmonella* spp., *Clostridium difficile* and *Shigella* spp. Where available, the ability to identify toxins from *Clostridium difficile* is valuable. Recently, the importance of looking for *Escherichia coli* 157 in patients with bloody diarrhoea has been recognized, and patients who have returned from under-developed countries may need investigation for other pathogens such as cholera.

Manometry and miscellaneous tests

Manometry

Oesophageal manometry has been an interesting development in the investigation of oesophageal dysfunction such as dysphagia and in particular chest pain of non-cardiac origin. Pressure is monitored using perfused tubes with side-holes which are attached to pressure transducers and placed in the oesophagus, but it requires much experience for correct interpretation. Achalasia is diagnosed by aperistalsis in the body of the oesophagus with impaired relaxation of the lower sphincter. Diffuse oesophageal spasm is associated with simultaneous non-peristaltic contractions of high amplitude and prolonged duration; repetitive waves and spontaneous contractions which are not induced by swallows are seen in many of these patients. Some centres with an interest in motility will perform anorectal manometry, and small intestinal manometry using telemetric pressure-sensing radio pills is being increasingly employed in the management of patients with motility disorders.

Oesophageal acid perfusion test

This is designed to establish whether retrosternal and epigastric symptoms are caused by abnormal reflux of gastric acid into the oesophagus. Perfusion is performed with the solution suspended on a drip stand behind the patient who is unaware of the nature of the perfusate. The test is positive if symptoms occur during perfusion with 0.1 M hydrochloric acid at 20 ml min^{-1} for 15 min but not during perfusion with saline at the same rate.

Gastro-oesophageal reflux studies

A pH electrode is positioned 5 cm proximal to the gastro-oesophageal junction and continuous monitoring is conducted over 24 h. If there is more than one reflux event per hour which reduces the pH to 4 or less, the test is positive. Furthermore, the length of time that oesophageal pH remains below 4 should be less than 10.5% of the time spent erect and less than 6% of time spent supine in normal subjects.

Pentagastrin test

Acid secretion is collected via a tube placed in the stomach with the patient lying on the left side. Following an injection of pentagastrin, normal peak acid secretion is $10-30$ mmol h^{-1} in women and $15-40$ mmol h^{-1} in men. In the presence of gastrinoma the basal acid output is at least 60% of the peak output after pentagastrin administration. Patients with duodenal ulcers tend to have higher acid secretion rates. Achlorhydria is commonly found in the elderly and is characteristic of atrophic gastritis which leads to pernicious anaemia. The value of this test has diminished with the development of more specific and less invasive techniques. However, surgeons still use the insulin stress test to assess the completeness of vagotomy. Gastric secretion is again collected via a nasogastric tube, the stimulus to secretion being insulin-induced hypoglycaemia. This test is unpleasant and can be dangerous if the patient becomes excessively hypoglycaemic.

Pancreatic function test

Intubation tests

These tests measure pancreatic exocrine function by analysing the duodenal aspirate after stimulating pancreatic secretion directly using secretin and cholecystokinin, or indirectly using a standard test meal. The indirect test is easier to perform but it will provide abnormal results in the presence of intestinal disease associated with impaired release of endogenous cholecystokinin, such as gluten enteropathy, as well as in primary pancreatic disease. In both procedures the tube is placed in the duodenum under fluoroscopic control to facilitate aspiration of pancreatic secretion. In severe exocrine insufficiency or with large neoplasms there is a reduction of the volume secreted as well as the bicarbonate and enzyme contents. Tumours compressing the duct will lead to a reduced volume of secretion with normal enzyme and bicarbonate concentrations. The sensitivity of these tests for the detection of chronic pancreatitis is approximately 80%.

Tubeless tests

The bentiromide test is based on measurement of para-amino benzoic acid in the urine or serum after oral bentiromide administration. This is not absorbed until it is cleaved by pancreatic chymotrypsin. A similar test is based on the absorption of fluorescein released by the action of pancreatic esterase on fluorescein dilaurate. Reference has already been made to the triolein breath test. Finally, many patients with pancreatic disease have an abnormal glucose tolerance test, but this is of no value as a test of exocrine function.

Hydrogen breath test

Hydrogen in the breath originates from the activity of intestinal bacteria on intraluminal carbohydrate. The measurement of breath hydrogen by hydrogen analyser is a useful and versatile technique. Excessive hydrogen excretion after a glucose load is indicative of bacterial overgrowth in the small intestine and after a lactose challenge suggests hypolactasia. The non-absorbed sugar lactulose may be used to measure transit time between the mouth and caecum.

Miscellaneous tests

The xylose test is still used to investigate malabsorption. Blood or urine levels are measured after a standard oral dose. This test lacks sensitivity; urine measurements are affected by impaired renal function. The alpha-gliadin antibody test has recently attracted interest as a potential screening test for gluten enteropathy. Antibody can no longer be detected in the blood following treatment with a gluten-free diet.

Diagnostic approach

This section tabulates the use of these investigations for the diagnosis of the problems outlined in Table 1.1; investigations are listed in descending order. Those given first should be performed on most patients. The investigations listed below are only undertaken when clinically indicated. *Most patients will not require all the documented tests.* However, it must be remembered that whereas primary investigations are needed to identify the underlying disease, secondary investigations may be required to establish the effects of the disease. Examples of secondary investigation include the search for evidence of anaemia in patients with ulceration or malignancy of the gastrointestinal tract, and the documentation of malnutrition in patients with Crohn's disease.

Heartburn

Consider: Peptic oesophagitis
Investigation: Endoscopy and oesophageal biopsy
                Inspect stomach and duodenum
                Haemoglobin if haemorrhagic oesophagitis
                24-hour ambulatory pH monitor, if not resolved by above methods

Chest pain (non-cardiac)

Consider: Oesophageal dysmotility
Investigation: Barium swallow
                Endoscopy for oesophagitis
                24-hour pH monitoring, or acid perfusion in few patients in whom diagnosis is obscure
                Oesophageal manometry

Dysphagia

Consider:	Peptic oesophagitis with stricture
	Oesophageal (or gastric) carcinoma
	Oesophageal web
	Achalasia or other motility disorder
Investigation:	Barium swallow
	Endoscopy (some would omit barium)
	Radionuclide studies
	Manometry—only if the above investigations have excluded the first three possible diagnoses

Anorexia

Consider:	General causes: drugs, depression, uraemia, hypercalcaemia, malignancy, alcohol
	Gastric carcinoma
	Liver disease
	Crohn's disease
Investigation:	Blood tests: full blood count (FBC), liver function test (LFT), urea, calcium
	Endoscopy and biopsy of stomach
	Intestinal radiology

Abdominal pain

Upper

Consider:	Peptic ulcer disease
	Gallbladder disease
	Pancreatic disease
	Liver disease
	Irritable bowel syndrome
Investigation:	Blood tests: FBC, LFT
	Endoscopy
	Ultrasound

Mid

Consider:	Small intestinal disease
	Aortic dissection
Investigation:	Small bowel radiology
	Ultrasound

Lower

Consider:	Large intestinal disease
	Disease of uterus, ovary or fallopian tubes
	Disease of the spine
Investigation:	Sigmoidoscopy
	Barium enema
	Colonoscopy (with negative or equivocal radiology)

Pelvic ultrasound (this may precede investigation of the colon in some patients)

Radiology of the spine

Vomiting

Consider: General causes: drugs, alcohol, raised intracranial pressure, uraemia, pregnancy

Peptic ulcer

Gastric cancer

Pyloric obstruction

Intestinal obstruction

Hepatitis

Pancreatitis

Investigation: Blood tests: FBC, LFT, urea and electrolytes (calcium and amylase when indicated)

Endoscopy

Plain abdominal X-ray

Small bowel radiology

Ultrasound of pancreas, etc.—this will precede barium study with suspicion of pancreatic disease

Diarrhoea

Consider: General causes: drugs, alcohol

Gastrointestinal infection

Irritable bowel syndrome

Inflammatory bowel disease

Colonic neoplasia

Malabsorption (see below)

Investigation: Stool microscopy and culture (and, where appropriate, laxative screen)

Blood tests: FBC, urea and electrolytes

Sigmoidoscopy

Barium enema

Small bowel study

Tests for malabsorption (see below)

Constipation

Consider: General causes: drugs, immobility, pregnancy, diet, hypercalcaemia

Irritable bowel syndrome

Colonic carcinoma

Investigation: Blood tests: FBC, others, including LFT and calcium when indicated

Sigmoidoscopy

Barium enema

Intestinal transit and motility studies

Gastrointestinal bleeding

Haematemesis and/or melaena
Consider: Peptic ulcer
                 Gastric erosions
                 Gastric cancer
                 Oesophageal varices
                 Mallory–Weiss mucosal tear
                 Haemophilia
                 Vascular anomaly
Investigation: Endoscopy
                 Angiography (rarely needed)

Rectal bleeding
Consider: Haemorrhoids
                 Polyps
                 Rectal or distal colonic carcinoma
                 Angiodyplasia
                 Meckel's diverticulum
Investigation: Blood tests: FBC
                 Sigmoidoscopy
                 Barium enema
                 Colonoscopy
                 Technetium scan
                 Angiography

Anaemia (iron deficiency)
Consider: General: poor diet, menorrhagia
                 Peptic ulcer
                 Colonic carcinoma
                 Inflammatory bowel disease
Investigation: Faecal occult blood
                 Upper endoscopy (if negative, distal duodenal biopsy—see
                    malabsorption)
                 Sigmoidoscopy
                 Barium enema
                 Colonoscopy
                 Small bowel study

Jaundice
Consider: General: haemolysis, Gilbert's syndrome, congestive cardiac
                    failure, septicaemia
                 Bile duct obstruction: gallstones, pancreatic inflammation or
                    tumour, bile duct stenosis
                 Hepatic: hepatitis, drug cholestasis, cirrhosis with
                    decompensation

Investigation: Blood tests: FBC, LFT; virology: hepatitis A,B,D,C

Prothrombin time; antimitochondrial antibodies (AMA), anti-smooth muscle antibodies (SMA), antinuclear factor (ANF) if indicated

Ultrasound—if in doubt about presence or cause of biliary obstruction, proceed to ERCP or percutaneous trans-hepatic cholangiogram (PTC)

If no dilatation—liver biopsy

Malabsorption and weight loss

Consider: Gluten enteropathy

Pancreatic exocrine insufficiency

Crohn's disease

Bacterial overgrowth

Short bowel syndrome

Enteric fistulae

Whipple's disease

Gastrinoma

Drugs: neomycin

Investigation: Blood tests: FBC, folate, vitamin B_{12}, calcium, prothrombin time, 25-OH vitamin D, alpha-gliadin antibody

Xylose absorption test

Faeces: fat excretion, microscopy

Jejunal (or distal duodenal) biopsy

Pancreatic function tests

Breath test: glycocholate or hydrogen

Schilling test

Small bowel study

Barium enema

Ascites

Consider: Hepatic decompensation

Malignancy—especially pancreatic

Cardiac failure—constrictive pericarditis

Meigs' syndrome

Investigation: LFT

Paracentesis: cytology, protein, culture

Ultrasound

Chapter 2
Respiratory Diseases

Introduction

The three cardinal but non specific symptoms of respiratory disease are cough, chest pain and breathlessness. No assessment is complete without a chest X-ray and some measure of pulmonary function. This chapter includes a summary of the major clinical features of respiratory disease, a review of standard investigations needed for preliminary assessment and the use of these investigations in common clinical situations.

Clinical symptoms and signs

A persistent cough may be a manifestation of bronchial asthma when sensitivity to non-specific irritants and nocturnal cough are characteristic. A nocturnal cough is also associated with gastro-oesophageal reflux and aspiration and such patients usually provide a history of heartburn. Nasal sinusitis with post-nasal drip and left ventricular failure with orthopnoea may also cause the patient to cough.

Haemoptysis is a potentially serious symptom which may reflect lung cancer, bronchiectasis, pneumonia or tuberculosis, as well as pulmonary infarction and mitral stenosis.

Breathlessness is very common. Rapid onset suggests asthma or pneumothorax; subacute onset dyspnoea is more likely to be caused by cardiac failure or pulmonary embolism; chronic dyspnoea is a feature of chronic obstructive bronchitis or emphysema.

Pneumonia may be acquired in the community. In previously healthy subjects *Streptococcus pneumoniae* or *Mycoplasma pneumoniae* are common pathogens, whereas those patients with chronic lung diseases may be infected with other organisms, including *Haemophilus influenzae* and *Branhamella catarrhalis*. *Staphlococcus aureus* is prone to infect patients with influenza and those suffering from cystic fibrosis. Hospital-acquired infections include *Escherichia coli* and *Klebsiella* spp.; anaerobes should also be considered following aspiration. Patients who are immunosuppressed suffer from unusual pathogens, including *Pneumocystis carinii*.

Pulmonary embolism may be heralded by breathlessness or pleuritic chest pain, pyrexia, tachycardia or a pleural friction rub. It should be considered in patients who are post-operative or immobile, particularly those with congestive heart failure or malignancy.

Pleural effusions are classified as transudates or exudates. Transudates (protein $<30 \text{ g l}^{-1}$) commonly occur in left ventricular failure and hypoproteinaemic states, such as the nephrotic syndrome or liver cirrhosis. Exudates (protein $>30 \text{ g l}^{-1}$) are found with local causes, e.g. malignancy, pneumonia and infarction.

21

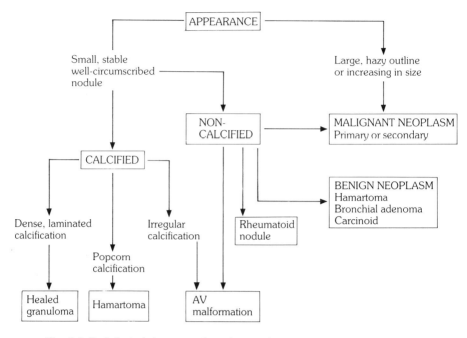

Fig. 2.1 Radiological diagnosis of a solitary pulmonary mass.

Bronchial carcinoma may present with respiratory symptoms such as cough or pleuritic pain, with weight loss or features of metastases such as lymphadenopathy, hepatomegaly or bone pain. Sometimes it is found incidentally as an opacity on a routine chest X-ray.

Abnormalities found on a chest X-ray require careful evaluation. The differential diagnosis of a solitary mass is outlined in Fig. 2.1 and of a pulmonary cavity in Fig. 2.2. Figures 2.3 and 2.4 respectively summarize the causes of diffuse pulmonary shadowing and a mediastinal mass.

The next section outlines the investigative techniques employed in the evaluation of patients with these clinical features or findings.

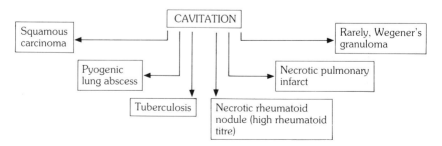

Fig. 2.2 Radiological diagnosis of a pulmonary cavity.

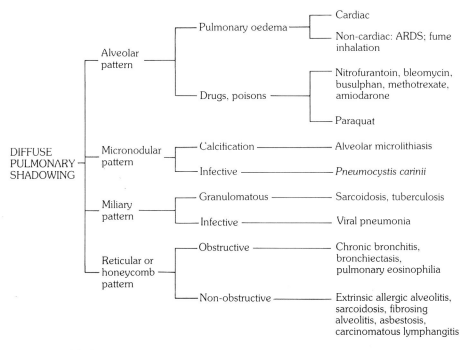

Fig.2.3 Some causes of diffuse pulmonary shadowing. Abbreviation: ARDS = adult respiratory distress syndrome.

Specific investigations

Radiology

The plain X-ray

The two views

The standard chest X-ray is a posterior-anterior (PA) view taken in full inspiration. This view is always to be preferred to a portable AP or supine radiograph as the latter are rarely of good quality and tend to magnify the size of the heart and mediastinum.

Lateral view

Important in the anatomical localization of an abnormality and especially good at displaying the anterior mediastinum and left lung base.

Oblique view

Valuable in displaying pleural plaques or for projecting lesions free of overlying structures.

Lateral decubitus view

The patient is radiographed on his side; the technique is useful in assessing

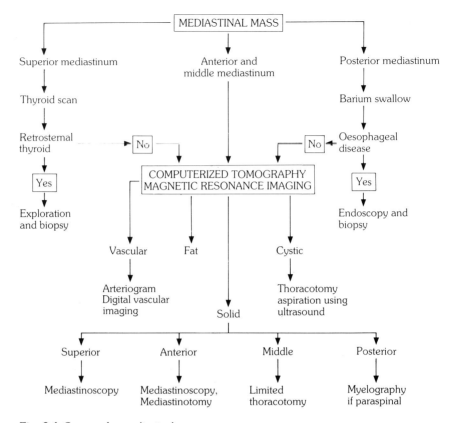

Fig. 2.4 Causes of a mediastinal mass.

subpulmonary effusions, fluid-filled cavities and the mobility of an intra-pulmonary mycetoma.

Expiratory film
Useful at demonstrating diaphragmatic movement, localized air trapping or a shallow pneumothorax.

Systematic interpretation
It is important that interpretation is done systematically, starting with basic information such as the name of the patient, date of film, projection and amount of rotation.

Trachea
Tracheal deviation indicates a shift in the upper mediastinum, e.g. from a collapsed upper lobe.

Spine
Scoliosis can make assessment of mediastinal structures difficult.

Mediastinum

A widened upper mediastinum may indicate lymphadenopathy or an aortic aneurysm.

Hilar shadows

Examine position, size and density of each hilum to avoid missing lobar collapse, tumour, lymphadenopathy or vascular enlargement.

Lungs

Follow the hilar vessels to the periphery of the lung as nearly all non-vascular shadows will be abnormal. Look behind the heart for a collapsed left lower lobe, seen as a faint oblique line from the hilum to the diaphragm, or a large hiatus hernia which may appear as a round shadow with a fluid level within it.

Heart

Look at the overall position, size and shape of the cardiac outline. The transverse diameter should vary between 11.5 and 15.5 cm. Examine each cardiac border for loss of clarity or additional prominence, especially below the aortic knuckle.

Diaphragm

The level, curvature and clarity of outline of each diaphragm should be noted. Flattening is usually a sign of obstructive lung disease. The margin of each diaphragm should be even and clearcut.

Skeleton

Remember generalized bone disease or localized abnormalities such as osteolytic lesions from metastatic tumour.

Difficult sites

Regions where lesions are most commonly missed are the apices, behind the heart and overlying the diaphragm.

The abnormal radiograph

Previous films may give insight into the evolution of a lesion.

Abnormal shadows must be analysed according to the anatomical site, size, shape and sharpness of outline, e.g. is the lesion localized and nodular or diffuse and reticular?

Segmental or lobar shadowing

A PA and lateral film will be required for accurate localization (Figs 2.5 & 2.6).

Is the abnormality due to consolidation, e.g. pneumonia; or collapse, e.g. bronchial obstruction from retained secretions or a bronchial carcinoma?

A collapsed lobe may be missed on a PA film unless other clues such as hyper-translucency or fewer vascular markings on the affected side are appreciated.

In the case of right middle lobe collapse, indistinctness of the right cardiac border may be all that is visible on the PA film.

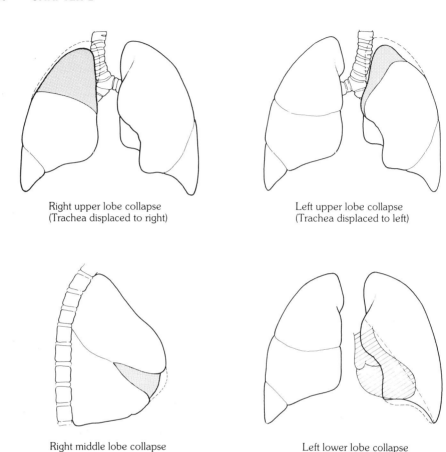

Right upper lobe collapse
(Trachea displaced to right)

Left upper lobe collapse
(Trachea displaced to left)

Right middle lobe collapse
(Lateral view)

Left lower lobe collapse
(Heart displaced to left)

Fig. 2.5 Characteristic PA (or lateral) appearances of lobar collapse. Displacement of trachea or heart may give clues to the diagnosis.

A left lower lobe collapse may be obscured behind the heart, especially if the radiograph is underexposed.

Computerized tomography (CT)

CT gives little additional information to a good quality radiograph in parenchymal lung disease.

Indications for CT

1 Examination of the mediastinum in the diagnosis of, e.g. aortic aneurysm, thymoma, pericardial cyst or lymphadenopathy.

2 The staging of malignancy by demonstrating local invasion or lymphadenopathy.

3 Detection of multiple pulmonary metastases including the pre-operative staging of those tumours that commonly metastasise to the lung, e.g. osteosarcoma.

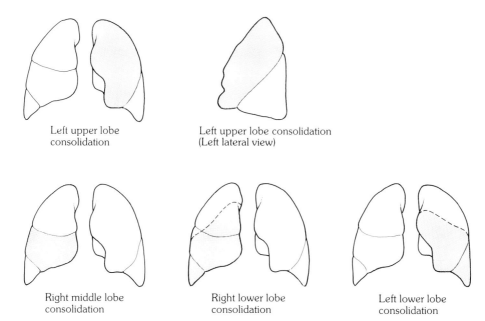

Left upper lobe consolidation

Left upper lobe consolidation (Left lateral view)

Right middle lobe consolidation

Right lower lobe consolidation

Left lower lobe consolidation

Fig. 2.6 Characteristic PA (or lateral) appearances of lobar consolidation. Upper lobe consolidation should raise the suspicion of tuberculosis or bronchial carcinoma.

4 Assessment of pleural disease including pleural mesothelioma and the differentiation of a loculated pleural effusion from a solid tumour.

Superior vena caval venography

The technique involves bilateral injection of contrast into the subclavian veins and is valuable in determining the site of superior vena caval obstruction and revealing unsuspected thrombus formation at the site of narrowing.

Pulmonary function

Every patient with lung disease should have at least one pulmonary function test and serial measurements are better. The limits of normality can be set by reference to the predicted value $\pm 20\%$. Patients suspected of having communicable respiratory disease, e.g. tuberculosis, should not have spirometry because of the risk of cross infection.

Patterns of abnormal pulmonary function are shown in Table 2.1.

Tests of ventilatory function

Peak flow

Patients are instructed to take a maximal inspiration and then exhale as forcibly as possible into a Wright's peak flow meter. Falsely low values can occur if patients are not encouraged to do their best. Accuracy is improved by taking the best of three efforts.

Table 2.1 Patterns of abnormal pulmonary function

	'Obstructive pattern'[1]	'Restrictive pattern'[2]	'Restrictive pattern'[3]
Ventilatory capacity			
FEV_1	↓↓	↓	↓↓
FVC	Normal or ↓	↓↓	↓↓
FEV_1/FVC	<70%	>80%	>75%
Lung Volumes			
TLC	Normal or ↑	↓↓	↓↓
RV	↑↑	↓	↓
Transfer factor			
TLco	Normal (asthma); ↓↓ (emphysema)	↓	↓
Kco (TLco/VA)	↓ (emphysema)	↓	Normal

[1] Airways obstruction, eg. asthma, chronic bronchitis and emphysema.
[2] Parenchymal lung disease, e.g. fibrosing alveolitis, sarcoidosis.
[3] Neuromuscular disease and normal lungs.

Ventilatory capacity

Ventilatory capacity is assessed by measurement of forced vital capacity (FVC) and forced expired volume in 1 s (FEV_1). The FVC is that volume of air that can be forcibly expired from the lungs between total lung capacity and residual volume. FEV_1 is that portion of vital capacity which can be forcibly expired in

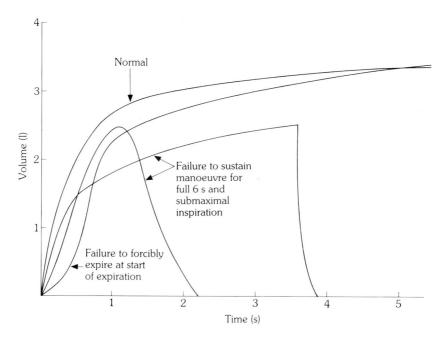

Fig. 2.7 Examples of some common errors seen during spirometry.

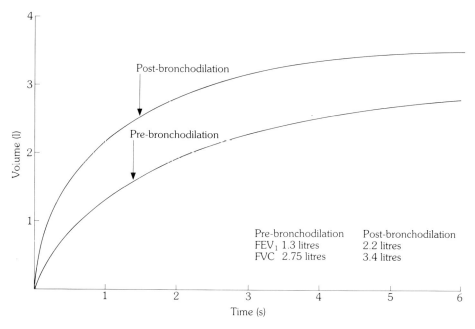

Fig. 2.8 Spirogram from a patient with asthma to illustrate the improvement following bronchodilation.

the first second. The ratio FEV_1/FVC expressed as a percentage gives a useful measure of airways obstruction, although poor technique poses problems (Fig. 2.7). Reversibility of airways obstruction can be tested by repeating the manoeuvre 10 min after inhalation of a bronchodilator (Fig. 2.8).

Flow–volume loop

The F–V loop relates instantaneous flow to the forced vital capacity. Measurement is the same as for the expiratory spirogram except that the expiration is followed by an immediate full inspiration to complete the loop. The F–V loop is of greatest value in detecting fixed or variable large airways obstruction, e.g. stridor due to retrosternal thyroid (Fig. 2.9).

Static lung volumes and capacities

More detailed study of lung function requires measurement of total lung capacity (TLC) and its subdivisions (Fig. 2.10). The TLC is either measured directly by body plethysmography or indirectly from the functional residual capacity (FRC) by the closed circuit helium dilution method.

FRC is sensitive to changes in either lung or chest wall compliance and FRC will increase with pulmonary emphysema and decrease with obesity or diaphragmatic paralysis.

Vital capacity may be reduced in both obstructive and restrictive lung disease and therefore is most useful when related to FEV_1.

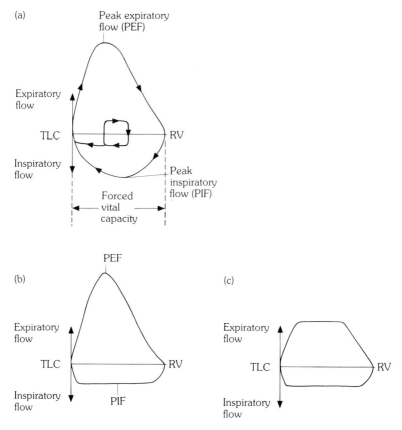

Fig. 2.9 The flow–volume loop in health and main airways disease. (a) Normal F–V loop. The patient performs a tidal breath and then inspires to total lung capacity (TLC) before making a forced expiration to residual volume (RV) which is then followed by a forced inspiration back to TLC. (b) Variable extrathoracic airways obstruction due to a subglottic tumour. The expiration curve is normal but on inspiration the extrathoracic airway narrows and airflow is restricted at the site of obstruction. (c) Fixed intrathoracic large airway obstruction—a more common finding that may be due to a malignant tracheal stricture.

Causes of reduced vital capacity
1 Airways obstruction from rise in residual volume.
2 Reduced lung compliance, as in pulmonary fibrosis or diffuse infiltrations.
3 Musculoskeletal abnormalities, as in myopathy or thoracic scoliosis.

Transfer factor

The transfer factor carbon monoxide (TLco) is usually measured by the single breath method in units expressed by the rate of uptake of gas from the alveoli in mmol kPa^{-1} of pressure difference between alveolus and capillary blood.

A low transfer factor may result from the following.
1 Loss of alveolar capillary bed, as in emphysema, pulmonary fibrosis or lung resection.

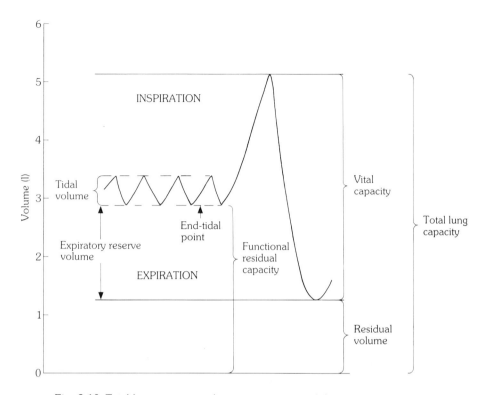

Fig. 2.10 Total lung capacity and its most common subdivisions.

2 Loss of pulmonary capillary bed, as in early collagen–vascular disease or pulmonary thrombo-embolism.
3 Reduced amount of haemoglobin (anaemia).
A high transfer factor may result from the following.
1 Asthma—due to increased pulmonary capillary blood volume.
2 Alveolar haemorrhage.
3 Polycythemia.

Exercise testing
This is useful as a challenge test in the diagnosis of asthma (Fig. 2.11).
The corridor walking test is a simple reproducible test which is used to judge the response to therapy. Patients are encouraged to walk as far as possible between two fixed points for a time period of either 6 or 12 min.

Blood gases
Blood gas analysis is essential in the management of acutely ill patients suspected of being hypoxic or in respiratory failure (Table 2.2).

Blood gas abnormalities

Causes of low P_{O_2}
1 Ventilation/perfusion mismatch leading to impaired gas exchange.

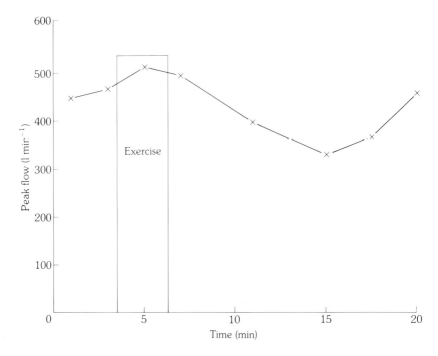

Fig. 2.11 Peak flow records before, during and after a bout of vigorous exercise to demonstrate exercise-induced asthma.

Table 2.2 Blood gas analysis and respiratory failure

Respiratory failure	Blood gas analysis	Causes	
Type I (V/Q mismatch)	$Pa_{O_2} \downarrow\downarrow$ Pa_{CO_2} normal	Moderately severe airways obstruction Fibrosing alveolitis Pulmonary embolism Pneumonia *or* pulmonary oedema	
Type II (hypoventilation)	$Pa_{O_2} \downarrow$ $Pa_{CO_2} \uparrow$	Sedation Acute neurological disease Chest wall trauma Scoliosis Chronic obstructive bronchitis End-stage lung disease	Often with an element of V/Q mismatch

2 Hypoventilation, as in ventilatory failure.
3 Cardiac shunts.
4 Reduced diffusion.

Alveolar or arterial Pa_{CO_2} tension is indirectly proportional to alveolar ventilation and is therefore an excellent indicator of ventilatory control.

Causes of low Pa_{CO_2} (hyperventilation)
1 Voluntary overbreathing.
2 Metabolic acidosis.
3 Hypoxic cerebral damage.

Causes of high Pa_{CO_2} (hypoventilation)
1 Depressed respiratory centre.
2 Failure of neuromuscular transmission.
3 Disorders of chest wall.
4 Inability of lung to respond to ventilatory drive, as in severe obstruction or end-stage fibrotic lung disease.

Peripheral blood examination

Blood count and sedimentation rate
1 Anaemia and a high sedimentation rate can be a non-specific finding in patients with malignancy, tuberculosis, severe infection or collagenosis.
2 Secondary polycythaemia usually indicates chronic hypoxia or carboxyhaemoglobinaemia from cigarette smoking.
3 Pulmonary eosinophilia is the combination of pulmonary shadowing and peripheral blood eosinophilia. This may take several forms, e.g. cryptogenic pulmonary eosinophilia, allergic bronchopulmonary aspergillosis, vasculitis, drugs (sulphonamides, nitrofurantoin) and parasitic infection.

Serum electrolytes
Hyponatraemia can indicate inappropriate secretion of antidiuretic hormone (ADH) by a small cell lung cancer.

The syndrome is confirmed by finding an inappropriately high urine osmolality in the presence of a low serum osmolality.

Serological test

Complement fixation tests
Useful in making a retrospective diagnosis of a pneumonia due to viral causes, *Mycoplasma pneumoniae*, *Legionella pneumophila*, Q fever, psittacosis.

Serum precipitins
Approximately 70% of cases with allergic bronchopulmonary aspergillosis have positive precipitins to *Aspergillus fumigatus*. Precipitins will be strongly positive in patients with an aspergilloma.

Inhaled organic dusts can result in a hypersensitivity alveolitis which is also associated with the production of serum precipitins (Table 2.3).

Positive precipitins always indicate previous exposure and are not absolute confirmation of the diagnosis.

Alpha$_1$ antitrypsin deficiency
An inherited defect caused by an autosomal recessive gene. This enzyme normally circulates in the blood and is a potent inhibitor of proteolytic enzymes.

Table 2.3 Examples of positive precipitins in extrinsic allergic alveolitis

Presentation	Source of antigen	Precipitins identified
Farmer's lung	Mouldy hay	*Micropolyspora faeni,* *Thermoactinomyces vulgaris*
Bagassosis	Mouldy sugar cane	*T. vulgaris*
Malt worker's lung	Mouldy barley or malt	*Aspergillus clavatus*
Bird fancier's lung	Pigeon, budgerigar, hen or parrot droppings	Serum protein

Its absence is associated with, severe, predominantly basal, panacinar emphysema presenting in the third or fourth decade.

Serum IgE
An elevated IgE level is strongly suggestive of an atopic predisposition.

Antigen specific IgE
There is an excellent correlation between skin prick tests and serum radio-allergosorbent tests (RAST) to most common environmental inhalant allergens.

RAST analysis is usually only considered when skin testing would be clinically unreliable or hazardous and only when the total serum IgE is raised.

Sputum
Early morning specimens are often best.

Inspection

Volume
Large volumes may be produced with bronchiectasis or lung abscess.

Smell
A strong, unpleasant smell suggests anaerobic infection as may occur with bronchiectasis or lung abscess.

Colour

Mucoid sputum
Clear and usually gelatinous in consistency. In asthma the sputum may be particularly gelatinous.

Purulent sputum
Yellow, brown or green sputum can imply secondary bacterial infection, although purulence in asthma may signify a high eosinophil count.

Melanoptysis
Black sputum is due to the breakdown of a coalworker's progressive massive fibrosis.

Microbiology

Gram stain
Gram-positive diplococci of pneumococcal infections and Gram-positive cocci of staphylococcal infections can be easily identified, although it is more difficult to distinguish *Haemophilus influenzae* from Gram-negative contaminants.

Gram staining is therefore more helpful in acute pneumonia than in exacerbations of chronic bronchitis, and is particularly useful when patients have already received antibiotics.

Culture
The most common pathogens isolated in respiratory disease are *Streptococcus pneumoniae*, *Haemophilus influenzae* and *Staphylococcus pyogenes*.

Gram-negative isolates usually indicate previous antibiotic therapy or nosocomial infection. *Klebsiella pneumoniae* or *Pseudomonas aerogenes* usually occur in previously damaged lungs, e.g. cystic fibrosis.

Candida albicans usually signifies oral contamination and is particularly common when broad spectrum antibiotics and steroids have been given.

Cytology for malignant cells
The chances of a positive result are improved by the collection of three good, separate specimens. Sputum cytology is more more likely to be positive for central desquamating tumours than for small peripheral ones.

Skin tests

The Sweat Test
In cystic fibrosis the concentrations of sodium and chloride in the sweat are raised. Values of sweat sodium concentration above 70 mmol l^{-1} are diagnostic of cystic fibrosis in children. In adults it is wise not to make a diagnosis unless the sweat sodium concentration exceeds 90 mmol l^{-1}.

Allergy skin tests
Allergy skin tests are used to determine the atopic status of a patient. There is no consistent relationship between positive skin tests and the aetiological agents responsible for asthma.

Most atopic subjects in the UK can be identified by their reaction to one or more of the following antigens: house dust; grass pollen; and cat (or dog) hair.

Kveim test for sarcoidosis

A 0.1 ml suspension of human sarcoid spleen is injected intradermally into the volar aspect of the forearm after first marking the site with sterile Indian ink. Regardless of the presence of a papule, the skin is biopsied with a skin punch at 6 weeks and is then examined microscopically for epithelioid cell granuloma.

Tuberculin skin test

Signifies hypersensitivity to tubercular protein and occurs approximately 4–6 weeks after infection with *Mycobacterium tuberculosis*. A positive result signifies a Type 4 delayed hypersensitivity reaction mediated by lymphocytes.

In clinical practice the tuberculin test is of limited value as it signifies both past and recent infection.

A *positive reaction* may occur with: active tuberculosis (strong reaction); following BCG vaccination; or previous infection with opportunist mycobacteria (weak positive).

A *negative reaction* signifies: no exposure to *M. tuberculosis*; or immunocompromised states brought about by old age, sarcoidosis, overwhelming miliary tuberculosis, malignancy or AIDS.

Bronchoscopy

The simplicity and safety of fibreoptic bronchoscopy under local anaesthesia has broadened the indications for bronchoscopy, and greater flexibility of the instrument allows more distal parts of the bronchial tree to be examined.

Fibreoptic bronchoscopy

Indications

Suspected malignancy

This is still the most frequent indication for bronchoscopy and suspicion will have been aroused by symptoms such as haemoptysis, stridor, unexplained cough, unresolving pneumonia or unexplained radiographic opacities. The majority of tumours will be accessible to direct biopsy or cytology brushings, but bronchial lavage or transbronchial needle aspiration of subcarinal lymph nodes is possible.

Diffuse lung shadowing

Bronchoscopy combined with transbronchial lung biopsy is now often employed in the investigation of unexplained diffuse shadowing due to suspected malignancy, granulomatous lung disease or unusual pneumonia.

Opportunist infection

When sputum cannot be obtained or may be misleading because of contamination with oral bacterial flora, fibreoptic bronchoscopy can be used to obtain specimens for examination either by bronchial brushings, broncho-alveolar

lavage or transbronchial biopsy. The latter can be useful in making
of *Pneumocystis carinii* or miliary tuberculosis, but in those with imi.
pression due to cytotoxic therapy or malignancy, better results can be at
with an open surgical biopsy.

Suspected bronchiectasis
Fibreoptic bronchoscopy provides a means for both bilateral and selective
bronchography.

Contra-indications
All contra-indications are relative but it is wise to avoid the following situations.
1 The uncooperative patient.
2 Where there is a likelihood of haemorrhage on biopsy, e.g. bronchial
adenoma, patients on anticoagulants, thrombocytopenia, superior vena caval
obstruction and pulmonary hypertension.
3 Poor respiratory reserve. Hypoxia often worsens during bronchoscopy.
Administer oxygen if the O_2 saturation is less than 85%. Naloxone or flumazenil
should be immediately available if sedation has been used.
4 Serious ischaemic heart disease. Bronchoscopy is best avoided for 6 weeks
following a myocardial infarction.

Specific indications for rigid bronchoscopy

Severe haemoptysis
Suction facilities are better.

Risk of haemorrhage
Where a tumour appears vascular, e.g. bronchial adenoma.

Staging of bronchial carcinoma
Surgeons may prefer to assess the operability of bronchial tumour by rigid
bronchoscopy as this technique enables them to 'feel' the extent of rigidity.

Photocoagulation
Provides improved access for laser therapy of bronchial carcinoma.

Bronchography

Patients with localized bronchiectasis can still benefit from surgery and these
patients will require bilateral bronchography to exclude generalized disease prior
to surgery.
    Selective bronchography via a fibreoptic bronchoscope may be helpful in
elucidating minor radiological abnormalities or in determining the cause of
haemoptysis when blood is oozing from a localized area of the bronchial tree.

Lung biopsy

Lung biopsy need only be considered if the radiological diagnosis is uncertain or the clinical setting inappropriate and where it is felt that a histological diagnosis will alter future management, e.g. steroid therapy. This may be obtained using a high speed trephine biopsy, or transbronchial lung biopsy at bronchoscopy.

To avoid complications the patient should have a normal platelet count and prothrombin time. Uraemic patients tend to bleed more and transbronchial lung biopsy is contra-indicated in patients with pulmonary arterial hypertension. About one in five cases will develop a pneumothorax and half of these will require intubation.

Fluoroscopy can help avoid haemorrhage from taking too central a biopsy and pneumothorax from taking too peripheral a biopsy.

Open surgical biopsy will involve thoracotomy but paradoxically may be safer in severely ill patients, especially if there is a bleeding tendency. It is used for the diagnosis of diffuse lung conditions where the disease might be patchy or in the diagnosis of serious infections in the immunocompromised. Specimens obtained are large enough for detailed histological staging and microbiological examination.

Diagnostic approach

Persistent unexplained cough

Most chronic coughs are associated with established disease such as bronchial carcinoma or chronic bronchitis, but there remains a small group of patients with a normal chest radiograph and spirometry who have a persistent unexplained cough (Table 2.4).

Table 2.4 Causes of unexplained chronic cough

Common
Bronchial asthma
Left ventricular failure
Main airway disease including inhaled foreign body
Diseased nasal sinuses

Uncommon
Laryngeal causes
Mediastinal tumour
Recurrent aspiration
Psychological cough*
Unsuspected bronchiectasis and cystic fibrosis
Drugs, e.g. angiotensin converting enzyme (ACE) inhibitors

* Psychological cough characteristically has a non-productive barking quality and the history will be one of several years, worse at times of stress (Fig. 2.12).

Haemoptysis

Haemoptysis must always be taken seriously, although in 40% of cases no cause will be found.

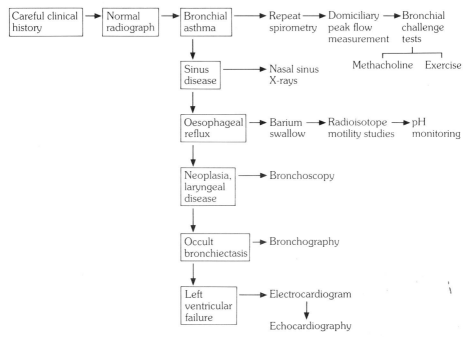

Fig. 2.12 Stepwise investigation of unexplained chronic cough.

The history should try and establish that the blood is truly expectorated and is not coming from the gums, oesophagus or nasopharynx.

Causes of haemoptysis are outlined in Table 2.5. A chest radiograph should form the basis of any planned investigation (Fig. 2.13).

Table 2.5 Causes of haemoptysis

Common
Chronic bronchitis
Bronchial carcinoma
Bronchiectasis or lung abscess
Pulmonary infarction

Uncommon
Pulmonary tuberculosis
Mycetoma
Mitral stenosis and/for pulmonary arterial hypertension

Rare
Bronchial adenoma
AV malformation
Clotting defects
Hereditary telangectasis
Goodpasture's syndrome

Breathlessness

Dyspnoea must be differentiated from hyperpnoea (normal response to exercise) and hyperventilation due to a metabolic or psychological cause. Shortness of breath is a very common respiratory symptom but most cases will be due to obstructive lung disease (Table 2.6).

Table 2.6 Some causes of breathlessness

Common
Airways obstruction
Left ventricular failure
Pleural effusion
Pneumothorax

Less common
Restrictive parenchymal lung disease
Valvular heart disease
Acute pulmonary embolism
Anaemia

Uncommon
Upper airways obstruction
Thyrotoxicosis
Chronic pulmonary hypertension (primary or secondary)
Neuromuscular disorders

Investigation

The following should form the basis of any planned investigation.

Haemoglobin

Anaemia
As a sole or contributory cause.

Polycythemia
Secondary or primary

Chest Radiograph

Lungs normal
Consider cardiac cause, pulmonary hypertension or neuromuscular disease.

Lungs abnormal
Neoplasia, diffuse lung disease or airways obstruction.

Pleural disease
Pleural thickening, effusion or neoplasia.

Disorders of thoracic cage
Disorders of the diaphragm, kyphoscoliosis.

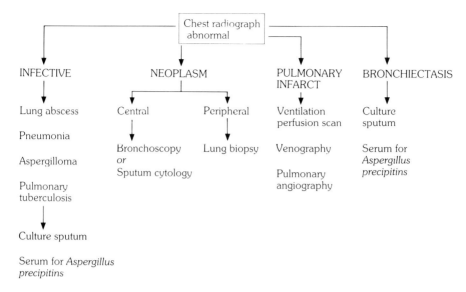

Fig. 2.13 Investigation of haemoptysis.

Lung function

Obstructive ventilatory defects

1 Fixed: emphysema (low TL_{CO}); chronic obstructive bronchitis (normal TL_{CO}).

2 Reversible: obstructive bronchitis (15–20% reversibility); bronchial asthma (>20% reversibility).

Restrictive ventilatory defect

Acinar lung disease (low TL_{CO}):

1 Sarcoidosis.

2 Fibrosing alveolitis.

3 Extrinsic allergic alveolitis.
4 Occupational lung disease.

Thoracic cage disorders (normal TL_{CO}):
1 Ankylosing spondylitis.
2 Kyphoscoliosis.

Neuromuscular disorders (normal TL_{CO}):
1 Guillain-Barré syndrome.
2 Myasthenia gravis.
3 Muscular dystrophy.

Detailed lung function

Maximal inspiratory ($P_{I max}$) and expiratory ($P_{E max}$) mouth pressures and maximum voluntary ventilation (MVV) identify respiratory muscle weakness.

Measurement of lung volumes and gas transfer factor should identify early cases of interstitial lung disease not apparent radiographically.

Flow–volume loop indicates upper airway obstruction.

Blood gases

Low Pa_{O_2}:
1 Ventilation/perfusion mismatch.
2 Hypoventilation.
3 Abnormal diffusion.
4 Right to left cardiac shunts.
Low Pa_{CO_2}:
1 Hyperventilation.
2 Hysteria.
3 Metabolic acidosis.

Exercise tests

Blood gases, minute ventilation and expired gases on exercise are a means of separating cardiac and pulmonary causes of dyspnoea and can be useful in identifying dyspnoea due to psychological causes.

Thyroid function tests

Breathlessness may occasionally be the presenting symptom of hyperthyroidism.

Isotope lung scanning

Ventilation and perfusion scans may reveal evidence of multiple pulmonary emboli as a cause of breathlessness.

Dynamic studies of cardiac function

Echocardiography or radionuclide angiocardiography may give evidence of a co-existing cardiac cause for dyspnoea.

Pneumonia

Chest X-ray
The following appearances can be helpful.

Lobar pneumonia
Typically pneumococcal.

Bronchopneumonia
Especially in old age or following aspiration.

Apical cavitating pneumonia
Consider *Mycobacterium tuberculosis* or fungal pneumonia.

Multiple nodular shadows
Typical of miliary tuberculosis or, if larger nodules, *Staphylococcus pyogenes* or fungal infection.

Diffuse bilateral shadowing
Cytomegalovirus or *Pneumocystis carinii*, particularly if of a perihilar distribution.

Pleural fluid
May indicate an empyema which should be aspirated and the fluid sent for culture.

Sputum

Gram stain
Gram-positive:
1 *Streptococcus pneumoniae* (diplococci).
2 Staphylococcus aureus (cocci).
Gram-negative:
1 *Haemophilus influenzae* (coccobacilli).
2 *Klebsiella* spp., *Escherichia coli.*
3 *Pseudomonas aeruginosa* (bacilli).

Culture
Gram-negative isolates should be taken as bronchial contaminants (especially post-antibiotic therapy) unless they are isolated repeatedly or in heavy growth.

Blood culture
Should always be taken in lobar pneumonia. Especially useful in diagnosing pneumococcal pneumonia.

Blood gases
Blood gas analysis must be considered in any patient with pneumonia as unrecognized hypoxia may lead to sudden cardiac arrest and death.

Pneumococcal antigen
Pneumococcal polysaccharide capsular antigen can be detected in sputum or any body fluid using counter immuno-electrophoresis. The result is highly specific and antigen may persist for 3–4 days, even in patients who have received appropriate antibiotics.

Further investigation if delayed response to antibiotics

Serology
Complement fixation tests on paired acute and convalescent sera can allow a retrospective diagnosis by showing a rising titre to, e.g. *Mycoplasma pneumoniae*, *Legionella pneumophila*, viruses, *Chlamydia psittaci* and *Coxiella burnetii*.

Bronchoscopy
In the non-immunocompromised, bronchoscopy will be directed towards excluding an obstructing lesion for lobar or segmental consolidation.

The immunocompromised host

Transtracheal aspiration
Using a sterile technique a cannula is inserted through the cricothyroid membrane and tracheal secretions are sucked into a syringe.

The technique prevents contamination of sputum by oral flora which is important because organisms that are normal commensals may be pathogenic in the immunosuppressed.

Bronchoscopy
1 Bronchoalveolar lavage.
2 Bronchial brushing. Useful for detecting acid-fast bacilli and fungal elements.
3 Transbronchial lung biopsy. Provides a means of diagnosing cytomegalovirus, *Pneumocystis carinii* and miliary tuberculosis and can also reveal underlying lung pathology, such as lymphoma.

Open surgical biopsy
The last resort, but often the safest procedure in severely ill patients or those with clotting defects.

Pulmonary embolism
Pulmonary embolism is potentially life-threatening and following immediate tests it is appropriate to anticoagulate with heparin whilst proceeding with further investigation (Fig. 2.14).

Immediate diagnostic investigation

Chest X-ray
1 Can be normal.
2 Oligaemic lung fields with massive pulmonary embolism.

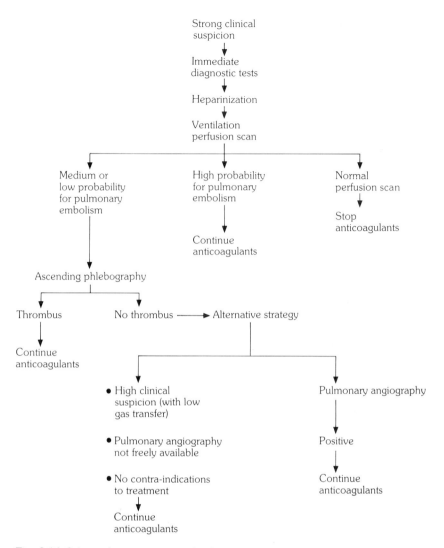

Fig. 2.14 Scheme for investigation of pulmonary embolism.

3 Elevated hemidiaphragm or small effusion.
4 Wedge-shaped opacities.
5 Linear atelectasis, especially post-infarction.

Electrocardiogram
1 Acute right heart strain.
2 Occasionally S_1, Q_3, T_3 pattern.

Blood gases
1 Hypoxia due to V/Q mismatch.
2 Hypocapnia from hyperventilation.

Ventilation/perfusion lung scan

Perfusion scan
Obtained by administering an intravenous injection of an isotopic complex of macro-aggregated human albumin tagged with technetium-99m. These complexes are sufficiently large to be trapped by the pulmonary capillaries and sufficient are given to produce a satisfactory image.

A *normal* perfusion scan taken in at least four views will virtually eliminate the diagnosis of pulmonary embolism.

An *abnormal* perfusion scan lacks specificity as many pulmonary disorders, e.g. pneumonia, emphysema and asthma can produce perfusion defects indistinguishable from pulmonary embolism.

Ventilation scan
Specificity is improved by simultaneously performing a ventilation scan. A radioactive gas (xenon-133 or krypton-81m) or suitable radio-aerosol, e.g. technetium diethylenetriamine penta-acetic acid (technetium-DTPA) is inhaled to build up a scintigraphic image of ventilation. Parenchymal lung disease is characterized by having matching ventilation and perfusion defects whereas pulmonary embolism causes a perfusion defect in the presence of normal ventilation.

Pulmonary angiography

An invasive investigation with definite morbidity and mortality but, nevertheless, the 'gold standard' for diagnosing pulmonary embolism.

Indicated for the confirmation of pulmonary embolism if lung scanning is indeterminate.

Used for the demonstration of a pulmonary embolism when surgery or thrombolytic therapy is contemplated.

Pleural effusion

Approximately 300 ml of fluid has to accumulate in the pleural space before it can be detected clinically or radiologically. Massive effusions usually indicate malignancy.

Plain chest X-ray

The radiographic appearance of a pleural effusion is characteristic (Figs 2.15, 2.16 & 2.17). A small effusion simply obliterates the costophrenic angle whereas a large effusion will show a homogenous opacity with a curved upper border. The chest X-ray may show an obvious cause for an effusion such as hilar enlargement from a bronchial carcinoma.

Pleural aspiration and biopsy

All patients with an undiagnosed effusion should have a pleural aspiration (Fig. 2.18) and if the fluid is an exudate, a pleural biopsy should be taken also.

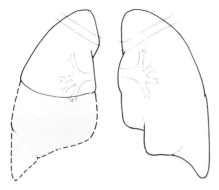

Fig. 2.15 Chest radiograph of a typical pleural effusion showing a homogenous opacity with a curved upper border.

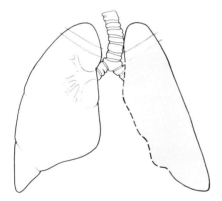

Fig. 2.16 Massive pleural effusion with marked shift of the trachea and mediastinum towards the side of the effusion due to tumour obstructing the left main bronchus and leading to associated lung collapse.

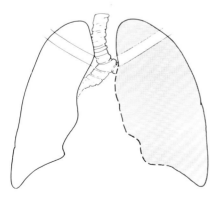

Fig. 2.17 Massive pleural effusion with shift of the trachea and mediastinum away from the effusion due to, e.g. metastatic tumour.

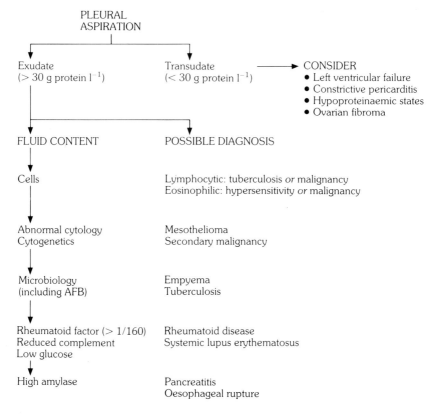

Fig. 2.18 Scheme for investigation of pleural effusion.

Complications

Pneumothorax
Due to inadvertent puncture of the lung or faulty connections in equipment.

Haemorrhage
Major bleeding usually indicates damage to an intercostal vessel. Pleural biopsy is contra-indicated in patients with clotting defects or those on anticoagulant therapy.

Pulmonary oedema
Often heralded by a recurrent cough which should serve as a warning sign. Probably caused by overzealous aspiration—restrict aspiration to less than 1.5 l at a time.

Pleural shock
A vasovagal reflex induced by pleural puncture or emotional apprehension or, more seriously, the occurrence of air embolism.

Analysis of pleural fluid
1 Protein content
   (a) Transudate <30 g protein l^{-1}.
   (b) Exudate >30 g protein l^{-1}.
2 Cytology
   (a) Lymphocytic (>50% lymphocytes): characteristic of malignancy or tuberculosis.
   (b) Eosinophilic (>10% eosinophils): non-specific, may indicate hypersensitivity or malignancy.
   (c) Reactive mesothelial cells: may indicate reactive pleurisy, as in pleural infarction.
   (d) Malignant cells and cytogenetics. Can provide a definitive diagnosis in experts hands.
3 Microbiology
   Fluid should be cultured for aerobic and anaerobic organisms. About 25% yield in tuberculous effusions.
4 Glucose
   (a) Reduced glucose concentration is non-specific.
   (b) Characteristic of rheumatoid effusions but also found with tuberculosis and malignancy.
5 Amylase
   Elevated pleural fluid amylase indicates pancreatitis, malignancy or oesophageal rupture.
6 Rheumatoid factor and LE cells
   Most rheumatoid effusions will contain rheumatoid factor but so will 40% of parapneumonic and 20% of malignant effusions.
7 Complement levels
   Connective tissue disorders can be associated with reduced levels of complement C_3 and C_4.
8 Haemothorax
   (Haematocrit >50% of peripheral blood): usually post-traumatic. Light blood-staining common in malignancy or post-pulmonary infarction.
9 Chylous or pseudochylous
   (a) Chylomicrons high and triglycerides >1.2 mmol l^{-1} indicates a true chylous effusion. Suspect lymphoma, metastatic carcinoma or trauma to the thoracic duct.
   (b) High cholesterol and lecithin globulin complexes indicates pseudochylous effusion. Found in chronic effusions or long-standing empyema.

Ultrasound scan
   Ultrasound is useful in differentiating fluid from solid structures and will allow guided aspiration of difficult or loculated effusions.

CT scan
   Very sensitive technique for differentiating between pleural fluid and pleural tumour. Especially useful in defining the extent of mesothelioma.

Fibreoptic bronchoscopy

Bronchoscopy can be helpful in undiagnosed effusions, especially if there is a history of haemoptysis or a hilar mass on chest X-ray.

Thoracoscopy and biopsy

If two attempts at pleural aspiration and biopsy have failed it is best to proceed to thoracoscopy as this allows direct visualization of the pleural surfaces with biopsy under direct vision.

Suspected bronchial carcinoma

Investigation

See Fig. 2.19.

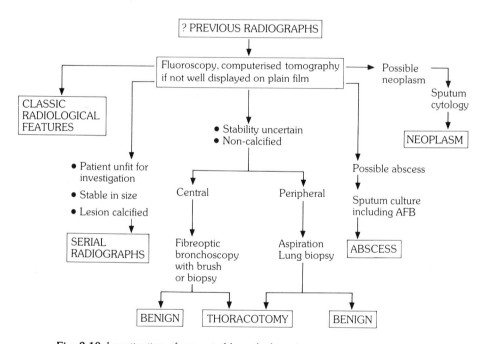

Fig. 2.19 Investigation of suspected bronchial carcinoma.

Assessment for surgery

Those remaining opacities of uncertain aetiology in patients who are potential candidates for surgery will need further assessment with regard to considerations such as age, lung function, cell type (central, small cell cancers are rarely operable), extent of local invasion and the presence of distant metastases.

See Fig. 2.20.

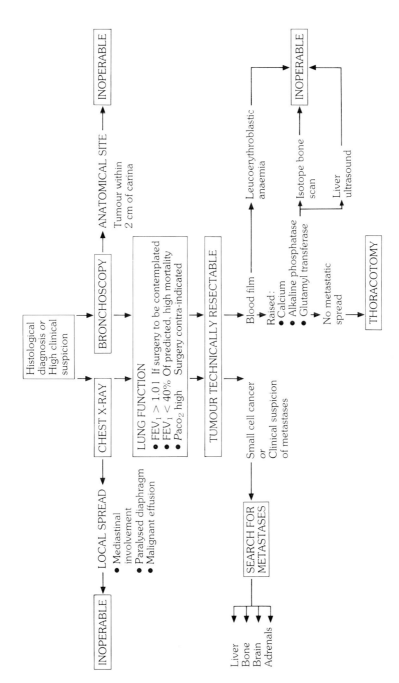

Fig.2.20 Pre-operative assessment of potentially operable bronchial carcinoma.

Chapter 3
Cardiology

Introduction

The main purposes of cardiac investigations are:
1 To confirm diagnosis of suspected heart disease.
2 To assess the severity of heart disease, and its effect on cardiac function.
3 Screening for heart disease.

General symptoms

Patients with coronary artery disease present with chest pain, typically a pressing retrosternal pain which may radiate to the jaw, back or left arm. Angina is usually provoked by exertion, especially after meals and in cold weather; it is relieved by rest. Atypical angina which may be associated with coronary artery spasm can occur at rest. The pain of myocardial infarction is usually more severe and prolonged, arises at any time and may be accompanied by nausea or features of cardiac failure. The latter features can herald myocardial infarction in the elderly who may not experience pain.

The symptoms of cardiac failure depend upon the predominance of left- or right-sided failure. Left ventricular failure presents dramatically with severe dyspnoea during which the patient prefers to sit upright and gasps for breath. Alternatively, presentation is more insidious with gradually worsening dyspnoea on exertion followed by orthopnoea and eventually paroxysmal nocturnal dyspnoea. The physical signs include a tachycardia (unless precipitated by inappropriate β-blockade or heart block) with a gallop rhythm and basal crepitations. Cyanosis may ensue. Right-sided failure is characterized by oedema, subsequently ascites and jaundice. The jugular venous pressure is elevated. Patients with heart failure may complain of non-specific lassitude.

Arrhythmia may be inconsequential, as with the palpitations that accompany over-indulgence, especially in coffee. Patients can be aware of paroxysmal tachycardia as a fluttering sensation which is sometimes followed by a diuresis. The development of atrial fibrillation in the presence of compromised cardiac function may precipitate cardiac failure. More serious arrhythmias, including extreme bradycardias or tachycardias, lead to transient impairment of consciousness or death; they can also provoke angina.

Specific investigations

Table 3.1 lists the main cardiac investigations, with the types of disease in which they are of most use.

Chest X-ray and electrocardiogram are the basic investigations which should be available in all cases of cardiac disease.

Table 3.1 Main cardiac investigations

Investigation	Disease*
Electrocardiogram	1–7
Chest X-ray	1–7
Exercise test	1, 6
Ambulatory ECG monitoring	1, 6
Echocardiography (including Doppler)	1–5, 7
Nuclear cardiology	1, 5
Cardiac catheterization	1–3, 5, 6
Electrophysiology	6

*1 = coronary disease; 2 = valve disease; 3 = congenital heart disease; 4 = hypertensive heart disease; 5 = cardiomyopathy; 6 = arrhythmias; 7 = inflammatory (pericarditis, myocarditis, endocarditis).

Electrocardiogram (ECG)

The ECG measures the electrical activity of the heart using electrodes applied to the body surface. Conventionally there are 12 leads, each of which is obtained by recording the difference in potential between two electrodes. These leads are given in Table 3.2. A normal 12-lead ECG is shown in Fig. 3.1. The ECG deflections are annotated by convention with letters and correspond to electrical activity in the atria (P) and ventricles (QRST) (Fig. 3.2).

Physiological variations in the ECG are important, e.g. in infancy, right ventricular dominance is reflected in large positive voltages over the right-sided leads (V_1 and V_2). Normal adolescents show generally high voltages which decline with age and obesity. Some ECG abnormalities are diagnostic of cardiac pathology (e.g. myocardial infarction), others reflect secondary cardiac effects (e.g. left ventricular hypertrophy) while others are non-specific, and their interpretation depends on a knowledge of the clinical setting (e.g. T-wave abnormalities).

Table 3.2 ECG leads

Bipolar limb	I	Right arm to left arm
	II	Right arm to left leg
	III	Left arm to left leg
Unipolar limb*	aVr	Right arm
	aVl	Left arm
	aVf	Left leg
Unipolar chest*	V_1	Fourth intercostal space to right of sternal border
	V_2	Fourth intercostal space to left of sternal border
	V_3	Midway between V_2 and V_4
	V_4	Mid-clavicular line, fifth intercostal space
	V_5	Anterior axillary line, fifth intercostal space
	V_6	Mid-axillary line, fifth intercostal space

* Unipolar leads are connected to an 'indifferent' electrode, formed by connecting all three electrodes, creating a 'zero' terminal.

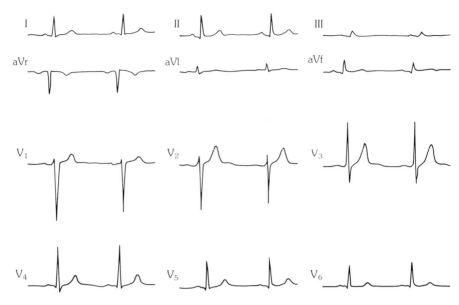

Fig. 3.1 Normal ECG.

ECG abnormalities

Arrhythmias
The ECG is an essential investigation in cardiac arrhythmias, with only a limited amount of information being obtainable from clinical examination. Variations in the normal P waves and P-QRS relationships are important, and may be best

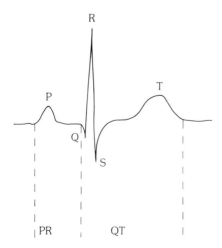

Fig. 3.2 ECG waveform. Abbreviations: P = atrial depolarization; PR = atrial depolarization + AV nodal delay, normally 120–210 ms; QRS = ventricular depolarization; T = ventricular repolarization.

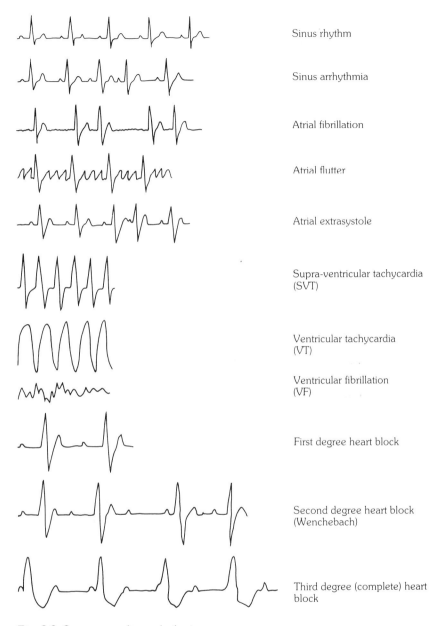

Sinus rhythm

Sinus arrhythmia

Atrial fibrillation

Atrial flutter

Atrial extrasystole

Supra-ventricular tachycardia (SVT)

Ventricular tachycardia (VT)

Ventricular fibrillation (VF)

First degree heart block

Second degree heart block (Wenchebach)

Third degree (complete) heart block

Fig. 3.3 Common cardiac arrhythmias.

recorded from leads II or V_1. Whenever possible, a 12-lead ECG should be obtained during an arrhythmia. Some cardiac arrhythmias are shown in Fig. 3.3.

Coronary heart disease
It is important to realise that the ECG can be normal in the presence of severe coronary disease. Myocardial ischaemia may cause ST depression, T-wave flattening or inversion. Myocardial infarction may be diagnosed by the presence

Table 3.3 The site of myocardial infarction

ECG lead	Infarction site
II, III, aVf	Inferior
V_{1-5}	Anteroseptal
V_{4-6}, I, aVl	Anterolateral
Tall R in V_1	Posterior

of Q-waves. ST elevation is usually found in the acute stages, along with T-wave inversion, changes which often regress. The site of infarction can be obtained by considering the leads showing the above changes, as summarized in Table 3.3.

Common cardiac arrhythmias are shown in Fig. 3.3. The changes of ventricular hypertrophy are illustrated in Fig. 3.4—in left ventricular hypertrophy the voltage in V_1 plus V_6 is at least 40 mV. Abnormalities of intracardiac conduction are shown in Fig. 3.5—in complete bundle branch block the RS duration exceeds 120 ms.

Electrolyte abnormalities
The ECG is a valuable method of recognizing potentially important electrolyte abnormalities. Hyperkalaemia is characterized by a decrease in the amplitude of

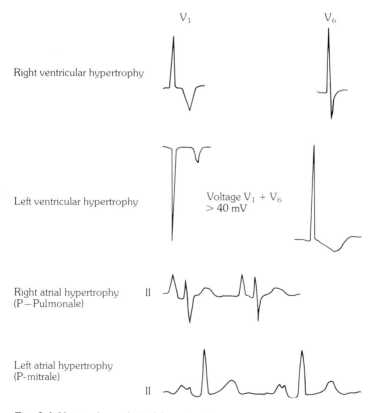

Fig. 3.4 Ventricular and atrial hypertrophy.

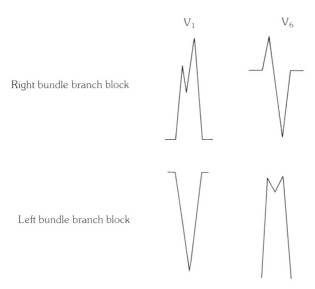

Fig. 3.5 Abnormalities of intracardiac conduction—bundle branch block (QRS duration >120 ms).

the P wave, tall peaked T-waves and QRS widening. Conversely with hypokalaemia there are prominent U-waves, T-wave flattening and inversion ST depression and PR prolongation. Hypercalcaemia and hypocalcaemia are respectively associated with a short and prolonged QT interval (Table 3.4). The ECG may also show characteristic changes with drugs, including digoxin, acute pulmonary embolism, pericarditis and hypothermia. These changes are summarized in Fig. 3.6.

The QRS frontal plane axis

Electrical activity can be represented as a vector, having both direction and dimension. All the components of a QRS complex can be arranged to give a mean vector, the direction of which is called the mean QRS axis. This is usually only measured in the frontal plane, using the 6 limb leads arranged on the 'hemiaxial reference system' (Fig. 3.7).

Table 3.4 Electrolyte abnormalities

Condition	ECG features
Hyperkalaemia	Tall peaked T-waves QRS widening Decrease in amplitude of P and R wave
Hypokalaemia	Prominent U-waves (after T-wave) T-wave flattening and inversion ST depression, PR prolongation
Hypercalcaemia	Short QT interval
Hypocalcaemia	Prolonged QT interval

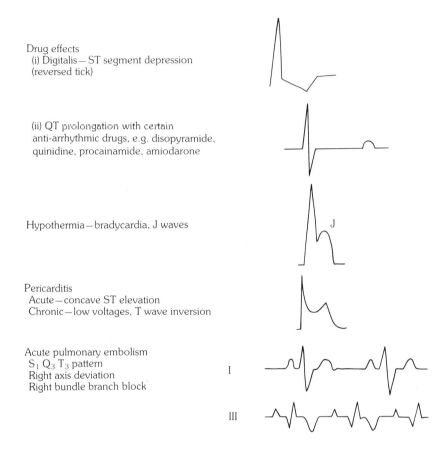

Drug effects
(i) Digitalis—ST segment depression
(reversed tick)

(ii) QT prolongation with certain
anti-arrhythmic drugs, e.g. disopyramide,
quinidine, procainamide, amiodarone

Hypothermia—bradycardia, J waves

Pericarditis
Acute—concave ST elevation
Chronic—low voltages, T wave inversion

Acute pulmonary embolism
$S_1 Q_3 T_3$ pattern
Right axis deviation
Right bundle branch block

Fig. 3.6 Electrolyte abnormalities resulting from the effects of drugs, hypothermia, pericarditis or acute pulmonary embolism.

To determine the approximate frontal plane axis, find the limb lead in which the QRS is most equiphasic. The mean QRS is roughly perpendicular to this; therefore look at a lead perpendicular to the equiphasic lead. If the QRS in this lead is positive, the axis follows the direction of that lead; if it is negative, the action is in the other direction. The normal axis lies between $-30°$ and $+90°$.

Calculation of the QRS axis is of value in several situations. Left axis deviation may be due to left anterior hemiblock, and right axis deviation may be due to left posterior hemiblock, and so in the setting of acute myocardial infarction change of axis may herald more serious heart block. Furthermore, the QRS axis may allow differentiation of ostium secundum atrial septal defects (right axis deviation) from ostium primum (left axis deviation).

Right axis deviation may occur in right ventricular hypertrophy and acute pulmonary embolism.

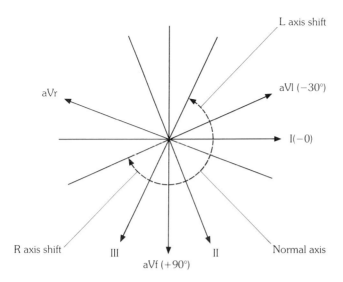

Fig. 3.7 The hemiaxial reference system.

Chest X-ray

Generally a postero-anterior (PA) film is taken, although a lateral film also yields important information.

The heart

A knowledge of cardiac anatomy is necessary to assess the various components of the cardiac shadow (Fig. 3.8).

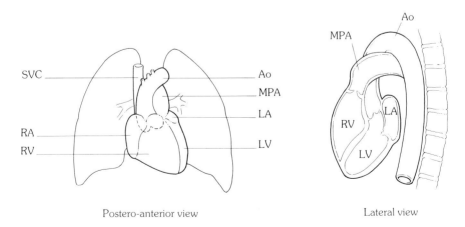

Postero-anterior view   Lateral view

Fig. 3.8 Components of the cardiac shadow. Abbreviations: SVC = superior vena cava; MPA = main pulmonary artery; LA = left atrium; RA = right atrium; LV = left ventricle; RV = right ventricle; Ao = aorta.

The cardiac shadow should not exceed half of the widest transverse diameter of the thorax, generalized enlargement may be due to generalized cardiac dilatation or pericardial effusion; in the latter, the heart shadow has a smooth and globular appearance.

Left ventricular dilatation as in mitral or aortic incompetence produces displacement and rounding of the cardiac apex. A bulge in the left side of the cardiac shadow suggests a left ventricular (LV) aneurysm. Left atrial enlargement in mitral stenosis is seen initially as a bulge below the pulmonary artery on the left heart border (atrial appendage). Later, a double right heart shadow is seen, and a lateral film, taken during a barium swallow, will show indentation of the oesophagus by the dilated atrium. Right ventricular and right atrial enlargement cause bulging of the right heart border and may decrease the retrosternal space.

The assessment of cardiac chamber size is now often carried out by echocardiography, although radiography remains very useful.

The demonstration of calcification within the cardiac shadow may indicate valvular disease (and is more easily seen on fluoroscopy). Pericardial calcification, suggesting constrictive pericarditis, may be linear or in plaques, and is often best seen in a lateral film. Occasionally, left ventricular aneurysms have calcification in their walls.

Dilatation of the aorta, with or without calcification, may be seen in the elderly, or in hypertensive subjects. Aortic aneurysm shows gross dilatation, and aortic dissection is suggested by progressive widening of the aortic shadow (there may also be a pericardial or pleural effusion).

Lung fields

Cardiac disease may lead to pulmonary congestion or pulmonary hypertension, both of which may be diagnosed from a chest X-ray.

The normal pulmonary veins are larger in the lower zones, particularly in the standing subject. With the development of pulmonary congestion (as in mitral stenosis and left ventricular failure), the pressure rises mainly in the lower veins, causing a reactive vasoconstriction and hence diversion of blood to the upper zones, with enlargement of upper zone vessels. Interstitial oedema produces blurring of the lower zone vessels and enlargement of the lymphatics, causing Kerley 'B' lines (horizontal lines in the periphery of the lung fields). Frank pulmonary oedema, as in acute left ventricular failure, causes fluid to collect in alveolar spaces, resulting in fluffy opacities in the mid and lower zones, and may cause opacities extending from both hilar regions ('bat's wing' appearance). Pleural effusions may be seen.

The normal pulmonary arteries decrease gradually in size towards the lung peripheries. In severe pulmonary hypertension, e.g. Eisenmenger's syndrome, there is enlargement of the central pulmonary arteries, but the peripheral vessels become small ('pruning'). In congenital conditions with left to right shunts, e.g. atrial septal defect, there is dilatation of the pulmonary arteries throughout the lung fields (plethora).

Inspections of the bony skeleton may reveal findings relevant to cardiac problems. Rib notching (inferior surfaces) occurs in coarctation of the aorta and sternal depression may cause cardiac displacement and a systolic murmur.

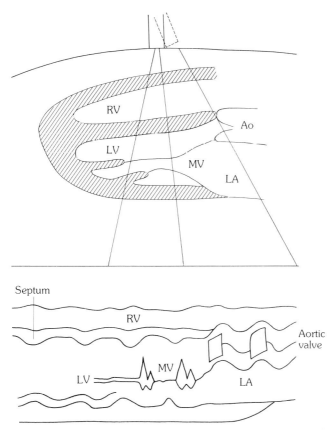

Fig. 3.9 M-mode echocardiography. Abbreviations: RV = right ventricle; LV = left ventricle; LA = right atrium; MV = mitral valve.

Echocardiography

The clinical use of ultrasound depends upon varying properties of the conduction of ultrasound in different tissues. There are two techniques for obtaining images of the heart: M-mode and cross-sectional echocardiography (CSE).

The original technique is M-mode echocardiography. Using a single crystal transducer, a beam of ultrasound is passed from the anterior chest wall (using the echocardiographic 'window' at the left sternal edge) through the heart, different structures being visualized by angulation of the transducer. The display is a moving record of cardiac motion, displayed on an oscilloscope and printed on moving paper (Fig. 3.9).

This technique allows accurate measurement of cardiac dimensions and precise timing of events, but only a small area of the heart can be studied at one time. Unlike other imaging techniques, the recordings are not recognizable as cardiac structures, and therefore considerable expertise is required in their analysis.

The technique of CSE is obtained either by rotating several crystals (mechanical sector scanner) or electronically oscillating ultrasound beams (phased array) and produces a two-dimensional 'slice' through the heart. This allows examination of the cardiac anatomy and is particularly useful in the study of congenital heart disease. By allowing the visualization of large areas of the heart simultaneously it provides information not obtainable by the M-mode technique, but measurements of cardiac dimensions and timing of cardiac events are less accurate. The two techniques are complementary and are usually used together.

Transoesophageal echocardiography using a transducer in a flexible endoscope allows very detailed examination of posterior structures, e.g. descending aorta or left atrium; it is particularly useful in the assessment of dissecting aortic aneurysms and prosthetic valve malfunction.

Uses of echocardiography

Valve disease

Mitral stenosis (Fig. 3.10)

The normal mitral valve leaflets appear as thin lines on M-mode echocardiography, and show a rapid diastolic closure rate of the anterior leaflet (EF slope), with the posterior leaflet moving in the opposite direction to the anterior. In mitral stenosis, there are multiple echoes from the valve (with dense echoes indicating calcification), a slow diastolic closure rate (flat EF slope), and both leaflets moving in the same direction.

CSE shows doming of the valve in diastole (caused by high left atrial pressure), and direct visualization of the valve orifice may allow calculation of the valve area (determination of severity of stenosis is not always reliable). Left atrial enlargement will be seen.

Mitral incompetence

Direct visualization of the mitral valve does not allow mitral incompetence to be diagnosed, and indirect evidence must be sought; this is mainly left atrial enlargement (not found in mild or acute incompetence) and a dilated left ventricle (volume overloaded). The cause of mitral incompetence can often be diagnosed:

1 Rheumatic; valve calcified, usually stenosed.

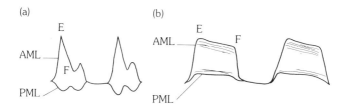

Fig. 3.10 M-mode electrocardiography of mitral valve leaflets: (a) normal; (b) mitral stenosis. Abbreviations: AML = anterior mitral valve leaflet; PML = posterior mitral valve leaflet.

2 Secondary to LV dilatation; LV poor contractility (contractility increased if incompetence is the primary lesion).

3 Myocardial infarction; may see flail leaflet (ruptured papillary muscle); ventricular dyskinesia.

4 Mitral valve prolapse; shown by systolic prolapse of one or both leaflets into the left atrium.

Aortic stenosis
Echocardiography will show thickened, possibly calcified, valve cusps, with restriction of valve opening (the latter allows differentiation from aortic sclerosis). In the younger patient with aortic stenosis the valve may not be thickened, but M-mode echocardiography may show a bicuspid valve (cusps eccentrically situated within the aortic root) and CSE may show doming of the valve in systole, with a small orifice at the cusp tips.

The left ventricle will be hypertrophied (with a small cavity size in the absence of aortic incompetence).

Aortic incompetence
As in mitral regurgitation, direct visualization of the valve does not allow the diagnosis of aortic regurgitation. A specific finding, however, is diastolic fluttering of the anterior mitral leaflet, caused by the regurgitant jet (the LV side of the IV septum may also be seen to vibrate). The diagnosis may be strengthened by showing the features of LV volume overload, i.e. dilated, dynamic LV (as in mitral regurgitation). In severe cases, there may be early closure of the mitral valve.

The underlying cause of aortic regurgitation may be found by echocardiography, for example:

1 Vegetations in endocarditis.

2 Dilated aortic root in Marfan's syndrome.

3 Calcification (rheumatic).

4 Double aortic wall (dissection)—not always seen on echocardiography.

The tricuspid and pulmonary valves can be visualized and stenosis or vegetations may be seen.

Myocardial infarction
The infarcted area of myocardium may show decreased contractility, akinesia or paradoxical motion. CSE may show the extent of the infarction and enable localization of the affected area. Unaffected myocardium may be assessed—hyperdynamic contraction may be present in such areas.

Complications of myocardial infarction which may be assessed by the technique include:

1 Ventricular aneurysm—a dilated, dyskinetic region.

2 Mural thrombus.

3 Mitral incompetence—flail leaflet, possibly LV or left atrial enlargement (often absent).

4 Ventricular septal defect—not usually visualized directly, but may be dilated RV.

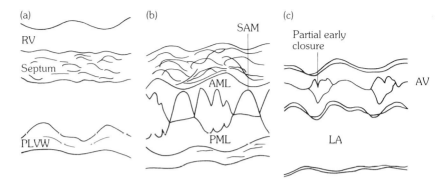

Fig. 3.11 Hypertrophic cardiomyopathy. Abbreviations: RV = right ventricle; PLVW = posterior left ventricular wall; SAM = systolic anterior motion; AML = anterior mitral leaflet; PML = posterior mitral leaflet; AV = aortic valve; LA = left atrium.

Other myocardial disease

Measurement of LV wall thickness is useful in diagnosis of left ventricular hypertrophy.

The ability to accurately measure LV dimensions and to assess myocardial contractility is very useful in the study of cardiomyopathies. In congestive cardiomyopathy, a dilated, poorly contracting left ventricle is seen—the global dysfunction in this condition may be differentiated from the regional abnormalities typical of ischaemic heart disease.

Hypertrophic cardiomyopathy (Fig. 3.11) has several characteristic features:

1 Asymmetric septal hypertrophy is the most constant feature; the septum is disproportionately thicker than the posterior LV wall. Septal contractility is usually diminished. CSE shows the thick septum and may show intramyocardial 'speckling', which may be due to the myocardial fibre disarray, typical of the condition.

2 Systolic anterior motion of the anterior mitral leaflet.

3 Partial early closure of the aortic valve.

The last two findings may indicate LV outflow tract obstruction.

Restrictive cardiomyopathy, e.g. as in cardiac amyloid, characteristically has a small LV cavity, ventricular hypertrophy and impaired contractility. High intensity myocardial echoes have been described in amyloidosis.

Congenital heart disease

CSE has greatly improved the ability to investigate congenital heart disease in infants and children, and in many cases cardiac catheterization is not now required. The technique is especially useful in delineating the anatomy of complex cardiac lesions, including Fallot's tetralogy and transposition of the great arteries. Contrast echocardiography, the formation of 'microbubbles' in the circulation by the rapid intravenous injection of saline or dextrose, can be used to visualize cardiac shunts, although this has a limited use. In adults, the lesions which can usefully be assessed are:

1 Atrial septal defect (ASD). M-mode echocardiography may show a dilated RV with paradoxical septal motion (anteriorly in systole), indicative of RV volume overload. CSE may allow visualization of the defect and allow differentiation of ostium primum and secundum defects.

2 Ventricular septal defect (VSD). This may be visualized by CSE, mainly when occurring in the membranous septum. Muscular defects are much more difficult to see. Enlargement of RV, LV and LA may be seen, although not in small VSDs. Contrast echocardiography may be helpful, especially if the shunt is from right to left (as in Eisenmenger's syndrome, where bubbles are seen to cross from RV to LV), although a negative contrast study (indentation of bubbles in RV by blood from LV) may be seen in a left to right shunt. The diagnosis of VSD by echocardiography is not always reliable (see Doppler ultrasound).

3 Patent ductus arteriosus (PDA). This may be visualized by CSE, but this is often difficult in adults. LA enlargement due to increased pulmonary blood flow is often seen.

Congenital valve lesions, e.g. biscuspid aortic valve may be diagnosed, although the pulmonary valve is less easily seen in adults.

Pericardial disease

One of the first uses of echocardiography was in the detection of pericardial effusion, for which it is the investigation of choice. An echo-free space will be seen in front and behind the heart and rough quantification of the effusion is possible.

Constrictive pericarditis may be deduced if, in addition to clinical suspicion, there is thickening of the pericardium with flattening of the mid- and late-diastolic motion of the posterior LV wall. Rapid closure of the mitral valve may also be seen. However, none of these signs are pathognomonic for constriction, hence the emphasis on prior clinical assessment.

Cardiac tumours

These are often well-visualized, especially left atrial myxoma, the commonest, for which this is the investigation of choice. CSE allows direct visualization of the tumour and is useful not only in diagnosis, but also in follow-up of the treated patient.

Endocarditis

A request for echocardiography to confirm or exclude vegetations is a very common reason for referral. Although the vegetations can be visualized, several constraints must be emphasized:

1 Small vegetations may not be seen.

2 Vegetations from previous endocarditis cannot be differentiated from actively infected lesions.

3 The most common problem arises in patients with pre-existing valve abnormalities, e.g. aortic sclerosis or stenosis, mitral stenosis, or with prosthetic valves. Under these circumstances, the valve and surrounding structures already show thickening, and it may not be possible to differentiate this from a vegetation unless previous recordings are available for comparison (routine post-operative

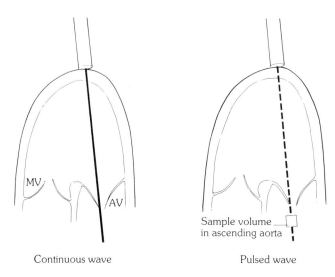

Continuous wave   Pulsed wave

Fig. 3.12 Apical long axis view of LV, mitral and aortic valves.

echocardiography of patients with valve replacement is very useful), or the vegetations are large and mobile. As well as showing the vegetations, the technique is, of course, very helpful in assessing the secondary haemodynamic effects of valve dysfunction.

Doppler ultrasound

This technique has come to prominence in the last 10 years, and now forms an integral part of every echocardiographic examination. The shift in ultrasound frequency detected by the Doppler mode is related to the velocity of blood flow, which can be calculated. The modes of Doppler ultrasound (Fig. 3.12) are as follows.

Continuous wave
This mode uses two crystals as one transducer—one to transmit and one to receive. It allows very high velocities (e.g. over stenotic valves) to be recorded but localization of the exact source of the signal (i.e. the distance from the transducer) is not possible.

Pulsed wave
One crystal both transmits and receives the signal; therefore some of the time is spent transmitting and some receiving. It is possible to select a small area for study (the 'sample volume'), thus enabling more accurate localization of the blood flow being studied. This mode is, however, limited by being unable to record high velocities.

Colour flow Doppler
This relatively recent development provides a colour display of blood flow using a colour representation of many sampling sites—flow towards the transducer is

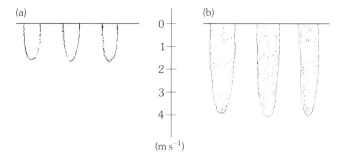

Fig. 3.13 Flow in ascending aorta from apical transducer position (flow away from transducer, i.e. below baseline). (a) Normal velocity 1.6 m s^{-1} (laminar flow). (b) Velocity 4 m s^{-1} (turbulent flow), i.e. increased velocity indicates stenosed aortic valve.

shown in red and flow away from the transducer in blue. Turbulent blood flow can be displayed in other colours, e.g. green. The scope of this technique is being assessed, but it is likely to be very important, particularly in congenital and valvular heart disease.

Applications of Doppler

Valvular disease

This technique allows accurate measurement of pressure gradients across valves, by measuring changes in velocity over the valve: the greater the increase in velocity, the narrower the valve. It is possible to calculate valve area from the change in velocity and this has shown good correlation with catheter findings in several studies. The continuous wave (CW) mode is particularly useful in stenotic valves (Fig. 3.13).

It is important to consider the *change* in velocity across the valve to assess pressure gradient; if the velocity below the valve is already high, then obviously a high velocity above the valve may not be due to valve stenosis (e.g. in hypertrophic cardiomyopathy the blood velocity is increased *before* the valve).

Valve incompetence is very reliably detected by Doppler; it is very well shown by colour Doppler. Although quantification of the degree of incompetence may not be very precise a rough estimation is certainly possible (Fig. 3.14).

Congenital heart disease

Doppler, in particular colour flow mapping (Fig. 3.15), is now a very important part of the echocardiographic examination of these patients. Flow through atrial and ventricular septal defects and patent ductus arteriosus is usually visualized, although the quantification of the shunt may be difficult. The severity of coarctation of the aorta can be assessed

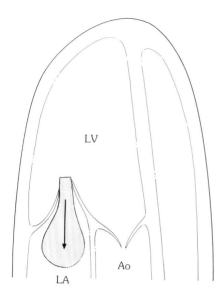

Fig. 3.14 Mitral incompetence period. Flow (from LV to LA, i.e. away from transducer) would appear blue on the colour display.

Nuclear cardiology

Radioisotopes have now gained widespread acceptance in the study of cardiac disease, especially in the study of coronary heart disease. Although many isotopes are under study, the two in widespread use at present are technetium-99m and thallium-201m.

Radionuclide angiography (RNA)

This provides a reliable assessment of LV function, both globally (ejection fraction) and regionally (wall motion analysis).

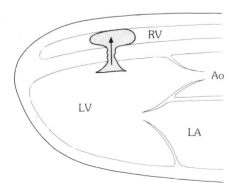

Fig. 3.15 Colour flow map—left sternal long axis view. Flow across a ventricular septal defect (from LV to RV, i.e. towards transducer) would appear red on the colour display.

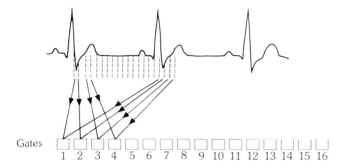

Gates
1 2 3 4 5 6 7 8 9 10 11 12 13 14 15 16

Fig. 3.16 ECG-gating in radionuclide ventriculography.

Equilibrium studies

The technique involves the labelling of either human serum albumin or, more often, the patient's own red blood cells with technetium-99m (^{99m}Tc) this prevents the isotope from leaving the blood 'pool' and therefore allows an outline of the cardiac chambers to be obtained. Serial studies can be performed over a period of several hours (half-life of ^{99m}Tc is 6 h).

Radioactivity is detected by a gamma-camera; however, as only a small amount of radioactive substance is given, the system is unable to resolve clear images over a single cardiac cycle. This problem is overcome by taking a number of cardiac cycles over a period of several minutes, by the use of ECG-gating (Fig. 3.16). In this technique each cardiac cycle is divided into a number of sections (gates), e.g. 16 or 32. Radioactivity from each gate is collected separately and combined to construct an average cycle, which is shown on a 'continuous loop' cine display.

These studies are performed at rest and can be repeated after interventions, e.g. exercise or drugs.

Information obtained includes:

Ejection fraction (EF)
This is the fraction of blood in the ventricle in diastole which is expelled with each systole, i.e. stroke volume/diastolic volume. The normal is >50%. Impairment of LV function will be reflected in a low EF, or a fall from normal on exercise (the latter commonly occurs in coronary heart disease).

Regional wall motion abnormalities
These include reduced motion (hypokinesia), absent motion (akinesia) or paradoxical movement. Regional abnormalities are suggestive of coronary disease, and again may be aggravated by exercise. LV aneurysms are well shown by this technique.

Myocardial perfusion imaging thallium-201

This isotope, an analogue of potassium, is extracted by healthy myocardium (by the Na^+-K^+ pump) after intravenous injection. Thus, uptake depends on both normal myocardial perfusion and metabolism, and abnormalities of either may cause absent or decreased uptake ('cold spots'). In practice, the main reason for cold spots is impaired perfusion due to coronary artery stenoses, although other conditions affecting myocardial metabolism can cause 'false' positives, e.g. cardiomyopathy.

Thallium-201 is injected intravenously at peak exercise, and maximal myocardial uptake is rapid. Exercise is continued for another minute and then imaging in three or four views (from anterior round to left lateral) is carried out, each view taking about 3 min to acquire. If defects are present at this stage (the patient is re-imaged some 4 h later) persistent (fixed) defects indicate myocardial infarction, while reversible defects indicate ischaemia.

The sensitivity of this technique in detecting coronary disease is about 85%, with a specificity of 90–95% (comparable with exercise testing).

Uses of myocardial perfusion imaging
1 Evaluation of atypical chest pain.
2 Assessment of radiographically borderline coronary artery stenoses.
3 Recurrent chest pain after coronary artery grafting.
4 Equivocal or non-diagnostic exercise ECG, e.g. bundle branch block.

Exercise testing

Useful information can be obtained from studying the response of the heart to stress; exercise electrocardiography is the usual technique employed. This is of use mainly in coronary heart disease, with information on some arrhythmias also being obtainable.

Techniques

Most protocols involve dynamic exercise, although isometric exercise, e.g. hand-grip, is also used. Originally, a simple two-step technique (Masters) was employed, with patients stepping up and down two steps; this has been superseded by treadmill or bicycle ergometer protocols.

Treadmill

The most widely used protocol is the Bruce protocol, which entails increments in the gradient and rate of treadmill. The advantages of using a treadmill are that walking is a familiar form of exercise, and that compared with a bicycle there is less dependence on patient motivation. Because of patient movement a satisfactory ECG may not always be obtained.

Bicycle ergometer

With this technique the patient's chest is stationary and a better ECG can be obtained.

Level of exercise

Exercise testing involves either maximal or submaximal levels of exercise. Maximal levels in the Bruce protocol are attained when the patient himself determines the end of the test, e.g. complaining of chest pain, dyspnoea or fatigue. This is the most commonly used technique. Submaximal exercise testing involves stopping the test after a pre-determined length of time or, more commonly, on achieving a pre-determined heart rate (often a percentage of the maximum heart rate predicted for the age group, which is obtainable from tables). This is often used in the pre-discharge test after myocardial infarction.

ECG lead systems

Many lead systems are available. Single lead systems have a sensitivity for the detection of coronary heart disease of 60%. More widely used multiple-lead systems, e.g. 12-lead, may increase this to 70%.

Exercise testing should be carried out under medical supervision, with full facilities for resuscitation, including a defibrillator, readily available. The overall incidence of ventricular fibrillation (VF) is less than 1 in 5000 tests. ECG recording and BP measurement is performed before the test, and at the end of each 3 min exercise level. Further recordings are taken at the end of exercise, and for 5–10 min thereafter.

Contra-indications to exercise testing:
1 Chest pain at rest.
2 Recent myocardial infarction (within 1 week).
3 Severe cardiac failure.
4 Severe systemic or pulmonary hypertension.
5 Aortic stenosis.
6 Malaise or pyrexia.

Relative contra-indications include:
1 Musculoskeletal disorders.
2 Exercise-induced arrhythmias, unless the test is being performed to investigate them.

Interpretation of the ECG on exercise is not possible in the presence of bundle branch block or digitalis therapy. Beta-adrenoceptor blockers should be stopped for 2–3 days before the test, unless it is designed to assess their effect.

Indications for termination of test:
1 End of exercise protocol.
2 Angina.
3 Exercise fatigue or dyspnoea.
4 Signs of peripheral circulatory insufficiency, e.g. pallor, clammy skin.
5 ST depression >2 mm, or ST elevation.
6 Hypotension.
7 Systolic BP greater than 280 mmHg.
8 Cardiac arrhythmias.

Indications for exercise testing

Coronary heart disease (CHD)

Exercise testing is useful in the assessment of patients with CHD. ST changes are the main findings, especially horizontal or downward-sloping ST depression (significant if greater than 1 mm at 0.08 s after the 'J' point). The test may be used after myocardial infarction to assess subsequent prognosis, using either a pre-discharge (submaximal) test or a late (maximal, symptom-limited) test, the latter about 6 weeks after the myocardial infarction

Assessment of atypical chest pain
Here the test is useful, but with important limitations. The sensitivity of the test is about 70%; therefore a negative test does not exclude the presence of CHD. The specificity of 95%, i.e. 5% of individuals with other causes for pain, will have a positive exercise test.

Study of arrhythmias
They may appear or disappear on exercise.

Ambulatory EGG monitoring
The ability to monitor the ECG over a period of time is extremely useful in the assessment of cardiac arrhythmias. 'Holter' monitoring allows tape recording of one or two ECG leads over a period of 24 h with a facility for the patient to mark, on the tape, the time of any symptoms, e.g. palpitations. The system enables selection and printouts of arrhythmias to be obtained. It is also possible to obtain counts of ectopic beats, heart rate trends and their relationship to arrhythmias (some equipment also allows analysis of ST-segment shifts, useful in the assessment of myocardial ischaemia).

The technique is useful in the diagnosis of arrhythmias, e.g. in patients with palpitations, dizziness or syncope, and also in assessing the affects of anti-arrhythmic therapy.

Cardiac electrophysiology (EP)
This is a very specialized procedure, available in a few centres, for the study of cardiac arrhythmias by recording intracardiac electrical activity with special recording catheters. The technique usually involves inserting several cardiac catheters, to measure activity in the RA, RV, His bundle and possibly LA (via coronary sinus) or LV.

Recordings are taken in sinus rhythm to assess cardiac conduction. Arrhythmias can be stimulated by pacing techniques, with or without extra stimuli; these techniques can also be used to terminate the arrhythmia once it has been studied.

The technique allows diagnosis of the mechanism of supra-ventricular tachycardia (SVT), with localization of accessory pathways, e.g. in Wolff–Parkinson–White syndrome; this can guide appropriate drug, pacing or surgical therapy. Ventricular arrhythmias are also studied, along with the effects of drug therapy. The site of initiation of ventricular tachycardia (VT) may be localized either by intracardiac (catheter) EP or at the time of operation by epicardial mapping, thus guiding arrhythmia surgery.

Simpler studies of sinus node and AV node function are possible, and can guide the need for pacemaker therapy.

Indications for EP
These include the following:

1 SVT: refractory to drug therapy, or where associated with major symptoms, especially syncope.

2 VT: refractory to drug therapy.

3 Survivors of cardiac arrest (unrelated to myocardial infarction): to assess inducibility of severe arrhythmias and the need for drug, pacemaker or surgical therapy (or more recently, an implantable defibrillator).

4 Sinus node and AV node dysfunction, if otherwise difficult to document, and if pacing is being considered.

Most patients with cardiac arrhythmias can be managed by therapy guided by clinical and ambulatory ECG assessment. Patients surviving cardiac arrest, however (when not associated with recent infarction), should probably always undergo EP study, because otherwise drug therapy is purely empirical.

Cardiac catheterization

As an invasive procedure, catheterization carries inherent risks. Careful consideration of the benefits likely to be obtained is necessary, and preceding non-invasive investigations may modify or even replace the procedure. Information gained from cardiac catheterization includes measurement of pressure, oxygen content of blood, cardiac output and assessment of shunt size and angiography.

The main risks are:

1 Damage to vessels, leading to haemorrhage, thrombosis or embolus.

2 Cardiac, including arrhythmias (common, usually self-limiting) and direct cardiac damage (rare, except in angioplasty).

Endocarditis following cardiac catheterization is rare, and prophylactic antibiotics are not routinely given.

Right heart catheterization

This is performed via a large vein (Fig. 3.17), usually the femoral or, less commonly, subclavian or cubital.

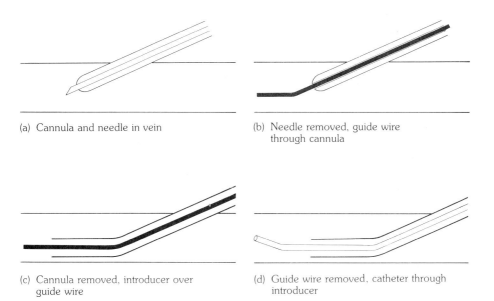

(a) Cannula and needle in vein

(b) Needle removed, guide wire through cannula

(c) Cannula removed, introducer over guide wire

(d) Guide wire removed, catheter through introducer

Fig. 3.17 Insertion of a catheter.

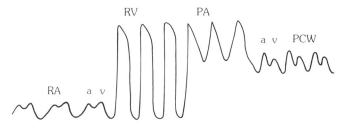

Fig. 3.18 Right heart pressure waveform. Abbreviations: RA = right atrium; RV = right ventricle; PA = pulmonary artery; PCW = pulmonary capillary wedge (equivalent to left atrial pressure); a and v waves indicate atrial pressure waveforms.

In patients with congenital heart disease, the catheter may take an abnormal course through the heart, e.g. through an ASD to the left atrium.

Pressure measurements

These are obtained through the fluid-filled catheter and via a transducer and are shown on an oscilloscope, as well as being recorded on paper (Fig. 3.18). Elevated pressures may be noted, e.g. in pulmonary hypertension, as may pressure gradients over narrowed valves.

Shunts

Shunts are assessed by measuring oxygen saturation in various sites, with the pulmonary : systemic (P : S) flow ratio being the main index of shunt size. This is calculated as:

$$P : S \text{ flow} = \frac{(\text{Systemic arterial} - \text{venous}) \, O_2 \text{ saturation}}{(\text{Systemic arterial} - \text{pulmonary artery}) \, O_2 \text{ saturation}}.$$

For an ASD or VSD, a ratio of greater than 2 : 1 is considered to merit surgical intervention.

Cardiac output

This is measured by various methods, but is not routine in cardiac catheterization. The methods all have the same basis which involves the mixing of a known amount of indicator with an unknown volume of blood. The Fick method is the one usually used in catheterization laboratories, and thermodilution, a simpler technique, is employed in bedside haemodynamic monitoring.

On the right side of the heart, angiography may be used to show right to left shunts, abnormalities of pulmonary circulation including pulmonary embolism, and to delineate cardiac anatomy in congenital lesions.

Left heart catheterization

This is performed either percutaneously via the femoral artery or via a cut-down on the brachial artery. The risks of haemorrhage and vessel wall damage are much greater in arterial procedures, therefore necessitating careful aftercare of the site. Patients on warfarin should have this withdrawn 2 days prior to left heart catheterization.

The catheter is fed retrogradely along the major artery to the aortic valve and across this into the left ventricle where pressure measurements are taken (the left ventricular end-diastolic pressure is a useful index which increases with the onset of impaired LV function). Angiography in the LV will show wall motion abnormalities and may reveal mitral incompetence or a VSD.

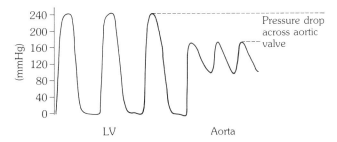

Fig. 3.19 Pressure waveform in aortic stenosis; withdrawal of catheter from LV to aorta.

The catheter is withdrawn across the centre valve, any gradient in systole being indicative of aortic stenosis (Fig. 3.19). Angiography in the ascending aorta will show aortic incompetence, aortic arch abnormalities, e.g. dissection or aneurysm, or coarctation of aorta.

Coronary angiography is carried out using specially shaped catheters, down which small quantities of dye are injected by hand. This outlines the coronary arteries and allows the visualization of atheromatous plaques; coronary anatomy, which is very variable, and the presence of collateral vessels are also important observations.

Diagnostic indications for cardiac catheterization

Valve disease
Stenosis of a valve is assessed mainly by measuring the pressure gradient across the valve when blood is flowing over it, e.g. LV to aortic gradient in systole for aortic stenosis (Fig. 3.19), or LA to LV gradient in diastole for mitral stenosis. A systolic gradient of 60 mmHg across an aortic valve or 40 mmHg across a pulmonary valve is usually an indication for surgery, as is a gradient of 10–15 mmHg across the mitral or tricuspid valve.

Valve incompetence is mainly assessed by angiography, when chamber enlargement and the incompetent flow of blood can be seen.

Coronary heart disease
Coronary angiography allows the visualization of coronary stenoses and the assessment of suitability for coronary surgery or angioplasty.

Indications for coronary angiography are as follows.

1 Angina refractory to medical therapy.

2 Angina following myocardial infarction.

Relative indications are:

1 Strongly positive exercise test (ST depression) in patients after myocardial infarction or with angina, as severe coronary disease is more likely.

2 Atypical chest pain, for diagnostic purposes.

3 During catheterization for other cardiac disease, e.g. prior to valve surgery.

Congenital heart disease

Catheterization allows the assessment of shunts, obstructive lesions, e.g. stenotic valves, and abnormal anatomy by both the passage of the catheter itself, and by angiography.

Procedures carried out by cardiac catheterization

Angioplasty

The dilatation of obstructive lesions with a balloon catheter can be used in coronary artery stenosis (percutaneous transluminal coronary angioplasty—PTCA). It prevents the need for surgery in some cases. Up to 10% may have serious complications from the procedure, e.g. coronary thrombosis, and facilities for urgent coronary surgery must be available; this means that the procedure is confined to major centres.

Dilatation of stenosed valves, mainly in congenital lesions, e.g. pulmonary stenosis, is undertaken in some centres although stenotic aortic and mitral valves are now also being treated.

Endomyocardial biopsy

In this technique forceps are introduced via the internal jugular vein. Biopsy of the RV may assist in the diagnosis of myocarditis, cardiomyopathies and cardiac transplant rejection (the latter forms the main use of this technique).

Suggested investigations

Angina pectoris

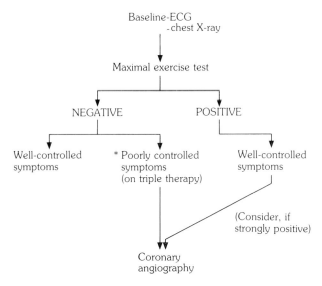

* Exercise test not necessary in this group.

Post-myocardial infarction (after discharge)

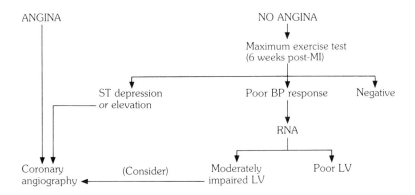

Arrhythmias

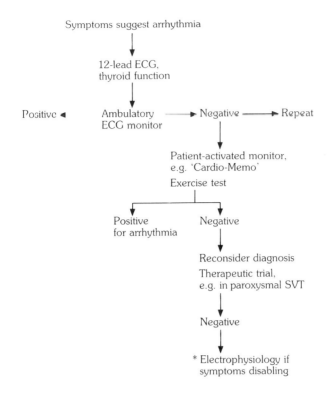

* EP testing is not often used to diagnose arrhythmias, but is more often used to guide the management of difficult, *already documented*, arrhythmias.

Heart failure

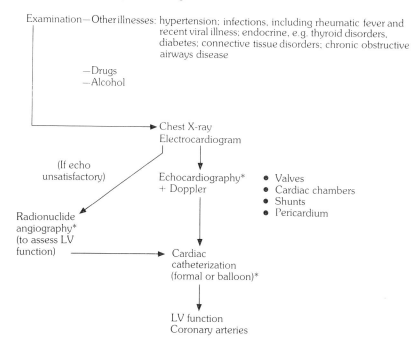

History—cardiac symptoms and signs.

Examination—Other illnesses: hypertension; infections, including rheumatic fever and recent viral illness; endocrine, e.g. thyroid disorders, diabetes; connective tissue disorders; chronic obstructive airways disease

—Drugs
—Alcohol

Chest X-ray
Electrocardiogram

(If echo unsatisfactory)

Echocardiography*
+ Doppler

- Valves
- Cardiac chambers
- Shunts
- Pericardium

Radionuclide angiography* (to assess LV function)

Cardiac catheterization (formal or balloon)*

LV function
Coronary arteries

*Also used in follow-up to assess effects of treatment.

Infective endocarditis

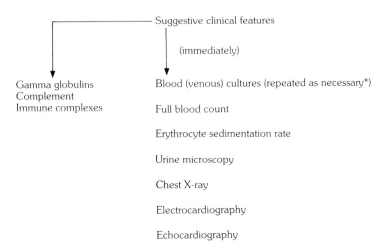

Suggestive clinical features

(immediately)

Gamma globulins
Complement
Immune complexes

Blood (venous) cultures (repeated as necessary*)

Full blood count

Erythrocyte sedimentation rate

Urine microscopy

Chest X-ray

Electrocardiography

Echocardiography

* Initial cultures negative, still strong clinical suspicion.

Repeat venous culture, also do arterial culture.

Treat empirically, awaiting results.

NB: In acute bacterial endocarditis, empiric therapy is usually started, once blood cultures have been taken.

Chapter 4
Arterial Disease

Introduction

Atheroma, a multifocal disease process, commonly involves the coronary, carotid and lower limb arteries. Smoking, diabetes and hyperlipidaemia are important contributory factors in the advancing atheromatous process. A careful history, examination and general medical assessment is followed by non-invasive vascular investigation using basic Doppler equipment. The need to progress to further investigation is dependent upon the patient's condition, lifestyle and the ability of any treatment offered to improve upon the natural history of the disease.

Symptoms

Symptoms depend upon which part of the vascular tree is maximally involved. Thus patients with coronary artery disease develop features of ischaemic heart disease including angina, arrhythmias and cardiac failure. Carotid artery stenosis leads to focal neurological symptoms, often culminating in a cerebrovascular accident. Narrowing of the lower limb arteries will cause pain on exercise, usually in the calf muscles, which is relieved by rest—intermittent claudication. As the process progresses the vascular supply is critically impaired causing pain at rest and, ultimately, gangrene.

Specific investigations

General medical examination

Routine vascular assessment should include a full blood count, erythrocyte sedimentation rate (ESR), urea and electrolytes, urinalysis, chest X-ray and ECG. Anaemia and polycythaemia will both aggravate the problem of vascular insufficiency and require correction. An elevated ESR may point to a vasculitis or inflammatory aortic aneurysm. Glycosuria suggests the possibility of diabetes. Many patients with vascular disease are smokers; thus the chest X-ray may show a bronchogenic neoplasm as well as an aneurysm.

Investigation of hyperlipidaemia

Cholesterol and triglyceride estimations are available in most centres, and are often sufficient for the management of such cases. Fuller analysis of lipoproteins may be necessary to allow classification of the hyperlipidaemia; the lipoproteins are listed in Table 4.1.

Exact classification of the hyperlipidaemia is not required in most instances, but is useful where available because it allows genetic studies and is important in

81

Table 4.1 Lipoproteins

Lipoprotein	Major constituents
Chylomicrons	Triglyceride
Very low density lipoprotein (VLDL)	Triglyceride
Intermediate density lipoprotein (IDL)	Triglyceride, cholesterol
Low density lipoprotein (LDL)	Cholesterol
High density lipoprotein (HDL)	Cholesterol

severe cases (Table 4.2). Although most cases of hyperlipidaemia are due to elevated LDL cholesterol, occasionally it can be caused by HDL elevation which is thought to be inversely linked with the development of atherosclerosis.

The most common types are II and IV, with familial hypercholesterolaemia being strongly linked with premature atherosclerosis (autosomal dominant inheritance; the homozygous form is uncommon).

For simple cholesterol and fasting triglyceride estimations the 'normal' values are: cholesterol $3.8-7.8 \, \text{mmol} \, l^{-1}$ triglycerides (fasting) $0.5-1.9 \, \text{mmol} \, l^{-1}$ (desirable cholesterol level is thought to be $\leq 5.2 \, \text{mmol} \, l^{-1}$). There is a tendency for serum cholesterol to increase with age.

Although most hyperlipidaemias are primary, other diseases can cause elevation in plasma lipid concentrations, and should be excluded in all cases. The main diseases are:

1 Diabetes mellitus.
2 Hypothyroidism.
3 Renal failure and nephrotic syndrome.
4 Cholestasis.
5 Gout.

Drug history (e.g. oral contraceptives) and alcohol intake must be assessed; the latter, if excessive, raises triglyceride levels (also HDL cholesterol).

Investigation of diabetes

Diabetes mellitus is associated with the development of vascular disease. The diagnosis of this condition is covered in Chapter 5.

Table 4.2 Hyperlipidaemia

Type	Lipoprotein increased	Cause
I	Chylomicrons	Lipoprotein lipase deficiency
II		
(a)	LDL	Familial hypercholesterolaemia
		Common polygenic hypercholesterolaemia
(b)	LDL, VLDL	Multiple hyperlipidaemia
III	VLDL remnants, IDL	Apolipoproteins 't' abnormality
IV	VLDL	Familial hypertriglyceridaemia
		Multiple hyperlipidaemia
		Common polygenic hypertriglyceridaemia
V	Chylomicrons, VLDL	Heterogenous group, including, lipoprotein lipase deficiency (plus other defects)

Lower limb vascular assessment

Non-invasive assessment

Ischaemia may be assessed by noting skin nutrition, capillary refilling and pallor or rubor of the limb depending on its position. Examination of pulses may indicate the site of an occlusion and the presence of a bruit 'a' stenosis. However, the distance a patient claims to walk before experiencing pain (*exercise tolerance*) is unreliable. Therefore, most patients should have a non-invasive assessment. In this respect, a comparison of the ankle systolic pressure to the brachial systolic pressure (*pressure index*) is recorded using a Doppler ultrasound probe, both at rest and in response to exercise. In health, the pressure index at rest is 1.0 or greater and during exercise will usually rise, whereas the ankle systolic pressure will fall in relation to the extent of the disease process. The recovery period necessary to return to the pre-exercise pressure index is a good indicator of the ability, or otherwise, of the collateral circulation to compensate. Where the recovery period is 3–5 min the collaterals are usually adequate, whilst progressive recovery periods beyond 5 min indicate a decompensating collateral system.

A further useful test with the Doppler probe is measurement of *segmental arterial pressures*, where a variety of specially designed blood pressure cuffs for ankle, thigh and arm are used. A suitable cuff is placed on the upper thigh and the systolic is recorded immediately below this level, the ipsilateral brachial pressure being the 'yardstick' of comparison, thus allowing pressure across the aorto-iliac segment to be recorded. A pressure difference of 30 mmHg or more, either across the segment or in comparison to an equidistant point on the contra-lateral limb, is significant. Cuffs are also placed above and below the knee and at the ankle, thus allowing pressure gradients to be recorded in the femoro-popliteal and lower leg vessel segments (Fig. 4.1).

If resting pressure indices are normal or near normal (0.8–1.0) and the exercise recovery period is within the 5 min, no further investigation is usually necessary, although the patient requires to be reassured and given general advice on smoking, diet, weight reduction and exercise. Where resting pressures are moderate to low (0.4–0.8) and the exercise recovery period is greater than 5 min, arteriography is usually advisable. With resting pressures of 0.4 or less, severe ischaemia is usually present. Pressure indices are, however, an arbitrary, and not absolute, guide to the severity of the disease.

Arteriography

Whilst adynamic and invasive, *arteriography* provides essential information regarding the nature and extent of the disease, allows definition of the state of the vessels above and below the lesion and displays the collateral circulation. In addition to conventional angiography, *digital subtraction angiography (DSA)* allows the option of an intravenous rather than intra-arterial delivery of contrast medium. DSA differs from conventional arteriography in that much smaller blood concentrations of contrast medium are required to produce diagnostically useful films. Before the constrast medium is injected, an image (the 'mask') is taken. After injection of the contrast medium, subsequent images have this mask

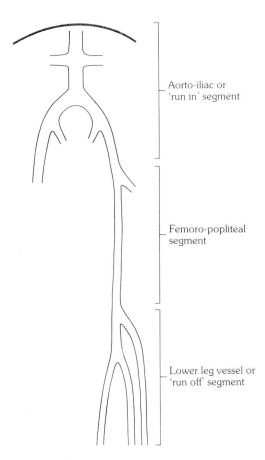

Fig. 4.1 Peripheral arterial segments.

(labels: Aorto-iliac or 'run in' segment; Femoro-popliteal segment; Lower leg vessel or 'run off' segment)

electronically subtracted, leaving a final image which demonstrates the contrast-outlined vascular structures free from background bone and soft tissue 'shadow'.

Upper limb vascular assessment

Upper limb ischaemia is a much less frequent problem with, more commonly, digital vessel involvement either by spasm, microembolism, arteritis or thrombosis. Where thoracic outlet compression is suspected an X-ray of that region may reveal whether a bony abnormality, e.g. a cervical rib, is present. *Arch aortography*, either conventional or DSA, will be necessary to delineate major vessel disease, particularly when unilateral. In those patients with suspected Raynaud's syndrome, the diagnosis is mostly made on clinical grounds alone, although measurement of finger systolic pressures and the vascular response to a cold challenge can help to clinch the diagnosis.

Internal carotid artery assessment

Examination of patients with suspected cerebral ischaemia may reveal the presence of a bruit over the carotid bifurcation, just below the angle of the jaw.

A bruit in this region may, however, represent a stenosis of the external rather than internal carotid artery, or it may be simply conducted up from the root of the neck. In order to establish the precise cause for the bruit, a non-invasive method of assessment should be employed in the first instance. These methods are many and varied, some with only limited value and an inability to distinguish between an occlusion or high-grade stenosis, e.g. *oculoplethysmography* or *supra-orbital Doppler* assessment: both are indirect methods.

Direct methods, such as *Duplex scanning*, are extremely accurate and should be used as first choice whenever possible. Pulsed Doppler, where the piezo-electric crystals are activated electrically for a short time, is used in imaging and allows visualization of the carotid or vertebral arterial tree in a biplanar fashion. This type of imaging also allows spectrum analysis of the wave forms obtained. Such is the precision of this technique that it is now more accurate than arteriography and avoids the need for arterial puncture in most patients. It is also particularly accurate in demonstrating the ulcerative plaque which has only a minimal degree of stenosis. However, when disease primarily affects the arch of the aorta, great vessels or intracerebral circulation, diagnostic arteriography is still necessary. In this context, intravenous DSA invariably gives poor results and *intra-arterial arteriography* should be employed unless there is a compelling reason for doing otherwise.

Aneurysms

Thoracic

Aneurysm of the thoracic aorta may be suspected on chest radiography, and the size and extent thereafter accurately determined by either an *ultrasound* or *CT scan*. *Aortography* may be necessary to determine accurately the involvement, or otherwise, of the origins of the great vessels or its continuity with the abdominal part of the aorta.

Abdominal

In 90% of patients the abdominal aortic aneurysm is below the level of the renal arteries, is pulsatile and palpable. Hence, the diagnosis is essentially a clinical one. *Aortography* is seldom necessary except when significant lower limb ischaemia co-exists and needs to be dealt with at the same time as the aneurysm.

Size (5 cm or greater) is about the only predictive factor which is related to rupture and thus, abdominal *ultrasound* or *CT scan* should always complement clinical examination. *Plain X-ray* of the abdomen will reveal evidence of calcification of the aneurysm in approximately 30% of cases.

CT scanning is particularly helpful in making the diagnosis of *inflammatory abdominal aortic aneurysm*, where the adventitial layer of the aneurysm may measure up to 1–2 cm in thickness. Although, if at all possible, inflammatory aneurysms should be operated upon, occasionally this is technically not possible, resulting in the need to put the patient on steroids. These patients are then regularly followed up by CT scanning until the inflammatory process abates sufficiently, as determined by the decrease in size of the adventitial layer, to allow surgery.

Chapter 5
Diabetes and Endocrinology

Introduction

This chapter reviews clinical investigation in diabetes and endocrinology. Diabetes is common, whereas many endocrine disorders occur very infrequently. Consequently, most emphasis is given to diabetes and an outline of the more important endocrine disorders.

The diabetic section follows the common format used in this text, whereas the endocrine disorders are considered individually, with a review of their clinical features followed by a summary of the more important investigations.

DIABETES MELLITUS

Clinical features

Diabetes mellitus is a syndrome characterized by hyperglycaemia. Two types of primary diabetes are recognized: insulin dependent and non-insulin dependent. Insulin dependent diabetes typically affects children and young adults. Plasma insulin levels are absent or low. It has an acute or subacute presentation, often with severe symptoms, marked weight loss and a tendency to ketosis. Non-insulin dependent diabetes mainly occurs in the middle-aged or elderly. Plasma insulin concentrations may be normal, low or increased. There is a more gradual onset with mild symptoms, or it may be a chance finding. Ketosis rarely occurs. Secondary diabetes is much less common. It is associated with destruction of the pancreatic endocrine function by disease or surgery, and with other endocrine disorders such as Cushing's syndrome or acromegaly.

Characteristic symptoms include polyuria, due to an osmotic diuresis associated with the hyperglycaemia and consequent thirst. The breakdown of muscle protein and fat leads to the loss of body weight. Patients with long-standing diabetes may have complications. Damage to the small blood vessels (microangiopathy) is most evident in the retina, with haemorrhages, exudates and new vessel formation which may cause loss of vision. Renal failure may develop due to glomerulosclerosis, for which proteinuria is an early hallmark. Diabetic neuropathy is most frequently sensory and affects the extremities. Patients complain of paraesthesiae or numbness. Motor neuropathy also occurs and is associated with muscle weakness. Occasionally some patients progress to develop autonomic neuropathy, with symptoms of postural hypotension, gastric distension and nocturnal diarrhoea. Diabetics are more prone to vascular disease such as ischaemic heart disease and peripheral vascular disease. Peripheral gangrene, typically affecting the feet, may arise because of a combination of impaired sensation leading to trauma accompanied by vascular insufficiency and infection.

Whereas all diabetics are advised to take a high unrefined carbohydrate and low fat diet in an attempt to minimize the blood glucose levels and delay the onset of vascular disease, insulin dependent diabetics require insulin replacement and many of the non-insulin dependent diabetics need oral hypoglycaemic drugs for symptomatic control. Insulin and some of these drugs can cause hypoglycaemia. The patient who is hypoglycaemic may have impaired consciousness, preceded by uncharacteristic behaviour, and has features of sympathetic drive, including sweating, pallor, dilated pupils and tachycardia. The hyperventilation and smell of ketones, which accompany ketoacidosis, are absent.

Specific investigations

The diabetic patient may require investigation to establish the diagnosis, to monitor diabetic control and to detect the development of complications such as retinopathy and nephropathy.

Examples of tests which are commonly performed during the everyday management of diabetic patients are shown in Table 5.1.

Some patients will also require more detailed renal and urological procedures, or neurological assessment. These techniques, such as renal biopsy and nerve conduction studies, are described elsewhere.

Blood tests

Blood glucose

Blood glucose can be measured by traditional laboratory methods or, more conveniently and rapidly, from capillary samples obtained by finger prick using test strips and a glucose colorimeter. Diabetics are taught to monitor the control of their diabetes by measuring the glucose values before meals and at bedtime in order to maintain concentrations between $4-10 \text{ mmol l}^{-1}$.

Random blood glucose

In a symptomatic patient a random venous whole blood glucose value of 10 mmol l^{-1} or more is diagnostic of diabetes and no further diagnostic tests are indicated.

Table 5.1 Examples of common tests required for the management of diabetics

Blood tests	Blood glucose
	Glucose tolerance test
	Glycosylated haemoglobin
	Insulin and C-peptide
	Urea and creatinine
Urine tests	Glucose
	Ketones
	Protein and microalbuminuria
Retinal investigations	Retinal photography
	Fluorescein angiography
	Ultrasound

Fasting blood glucose
Fasting venous blood glucose concentrations of greater than $7\,\text{mmol}\,\text{l}^{-1}$ confirms the diagnosis of diabetes; further diagnostic tests are not required.

Oral glucose tolerance test

A 75 g oral glucose load in 250 ml of water should be used in adults and loads of $1.75\,\text{g}\,\text{kg}^{-1}$ ideal body weight, to a maximum of 75 g, in children. Diagnostic criteria are shown in Table 5.2.

Table 5.2 Diagnostic criteria for oral glucose tolerance tests (glucose $\text{mmol}\,\text{l}^{-1}$)

	Fasting	2 h post-glucose
Diabetes mellitus		
Venous whole blood	$\geqslant7$	$\geqslant10$
Capillary whole blood	$\geqslant7$	$\geqslant11$
Venous plasma	$\geqslant8$	$\geqslant11$
Impaired glucose tolerance		
Venous whole blood	<7	$\geqslant7{-}10$
Capillary whole blood	<7	$\geqslant8{-}11$
Venous plasma	<8	$\geqslant8{-}11$
Normal		
Venous whole blood	<7	<7
Capillary whole blood	<7	<8
Venous plasma	<8	<8

There is a group with impaired glucose tolerance between frank diabetes and normality; 2–4% per year will become diabetic while a similar number will revert to normal.

Glycosylated haemoglobin

Glycosylated haemoglobin (HbA_1) reflects mean ambient blood glucose concentrations over the preceding 6–8 weeks, the half-life of the red cell. This is a valuable tool which is used to complement other methods of monitoring diabetic control. Results may be affected by conditions which shorten red cell survival; normal values range from 3–7% and 4–9% depending on the method of analysis.

More recently, serum fructosamine (principally glycosylated albumin) has been advocated for this purpose, as it is cheaper to measure. It also reflects mean values over a shorter time span.

Urea and creatinine

Serial measurements of renal function are an important aspect of diabetic monitoring. This is particularly important in the presence of proteinuria and hypertension.

Patients who are admitted in diabetic keto-acidosis require careful monitoring of their urea, electrolytes and pH.

Urine tests

Glucose

Traditionally, urine is checked for glucose as a screening test for diabetes or for the monitoring of diabetic control, using one of the proprietary stix tests. Glucose does not usually appear in the urine until blood glucose values reach $10 \, mmol \, l^{-1}$. However, some patients have a reduced renal threshold; this particularly applies during pregnancy. In contrast, the elderly and those with renal impairment have high thresholds. Measurement of glucose in the blood is more accurate.

Ketones

Ketones can be detected by stick testing during keto-acidosis and also during starvation.

Protein and microalbuminuria

Proteinuria is a pointer to the development of diabetic nephropathy. Dipstix methods are able to register traces of protein in the order of $50 \, mg \, l^{-1}$; the concentrated overnight sample is most likely to be positive.

Lesser degrees of proteinuria (microalbuminuria) may be detectable by radio-immunoassay. Microalbuminuria may also be caused by exercise or other intercurrent illness and these causes should be taken into account when evaluating the significance of a positive result.

Albumin excretion rates above $7 \, \mu g \, min^{-1}$ are abnormal. Heavy proteinuria ($>3 \, g \, day^{-1}$) strongly suggests diabetic nephropathy or co-incidental glomerulo-nephritis.

Retinal investigations

Retinal photography

This is an accurate way of recording the state of the retina and allows progressive changes to be monitored.

Fluorescein angiography

This consists of rapid sequence photography of the retina after the intravenous administration of sodium fluorescein. Early phase pictures show abnormalities of the microcirculation in greater detail and also demonstrate areas of capillary non-perfusion, which may be the substrate for subsequent new vessel formation. Abnormal capillary leakage is apparent from later phase pictures.

The injection may cause transient nausea; it leads to yellow discoloration of the skin, iris and urine.

Ultrasound

This is a useful technique in a minority of patients who have opacities in the media, e.g. those with dense cataract or vitreous haemorrhage, which preclude other methods of identifying possible retinal detachment.

Diagnostic approach

Hyperglycaemia

A fasting or random blood glucose value greater than $7\,mmol\,l^{-1}$ and $10\,mmol\,l^{-1}$ respectively in the presence of diabetic symptoms is diagnostic of diabetes.

High post-prandial glucose values may occur in non-diabetic patients who have undergone gastric surgery. Some patients have a low renal threshold for glucose so that glycosuria is detected during routine examinations; this particularly applies during pregnancy. Under these circumstances a glucose tolerance test is required.

Diabetic monitoring

Diabetics are monitored to ensure the adequacy of glycaemic control and to identify complications.

Diabetic control

Traditionally, patients were taught to check their urine for glucose and ketones. The wide availability of reflectance meters facilitates blood glucose measurements, which provide a more accurate assessment of control, particularly in patients with impaired renal function. Measurements are made before each meal and at bedtime.

Glycosylated haemoglobin is measured at routine follow-up as it provides an index of control over the preceding 6–8 weeks.

Complications

Nephropathy

Urine is checked for protein and albumin at 6-monthly intervals. If heavy proteinuria develops suddenly or in the absence of retinopathy, renal biopsy may be indicated to look for other forms of renal disease.

Blood urea and creatinine are monitored.

The investigation of possible diabetic nephropathy identified on the basis of these screening tests is summarized in Table 5.3.

Table 5.3 Investigations of nephropathy

Microalbuminuria
Proteinuria
  Intermittent
  Persistent
Urine culture
Urine microscopy
24-hour urine protein excretion
Urine protein selectivity (non-selective in diabetic nephropathy)
Plasma creatinine
Creatinine clearance
Renal ultrasound
IVU
Renal biopsy

Retinopathy

The retinae are inspected at review. The appearances which demand urgent referral to an ophthalmologist are summarized in Table 5.4.

Table 5.4 Appearances which demand urgent referral to an ophthalmologist

New vessels
Pre-proliferative changes (numerous cotton wool spots, venous loops, venous infarcts)
Hard exudates encroaching on the macula
Loss of visual acuity without obvious retinopathy (? macular oedema)

Retinal photography is used to accurately document progress.

Fluorescein angiography documents areas of non-perfusion and abnormal leakage.

Neuropathy

The development of neuropathic features may require neurological investigation as outlined in Chapter 6.

Hypoglycaemia

Spontaneous hypoglycaemia can be divided into two categories, fasting or post-prandial (reactive). The causes of spontaneous hypoglycaemia are given in Table 5.5.

Table 5.5 Causes of spontaneous hypoglycaemia

Fasting
  Insulinoma
  Hypopituitarism
  Addison's disease
  Hypothyroidism
  Liver failure
  Sarcoma
  Ethanol
  Factitious (administration of insulin or oral hypoglycaemic agents)

Post-prandial
  Gastric surgery
  'Mild' diabetes

Fasting hypoglycaemia is investigated as outlined in Fig. 5.1.

Techniques used to localize an insulinoma include coeliac axis arteriography, CT scan with angiography and trans-hepatic portal vein cannulation for retrograde venography and venous sampling for insulin.

Insulin and C-peptide

These measurements may be required in patients who develop hypoglycaemia of uncertain cause. If the insulin values are high, an elevated C-peptide denotes autonomous insulin secretion rather than self-administration with insulin when C-peptide is undetectable.

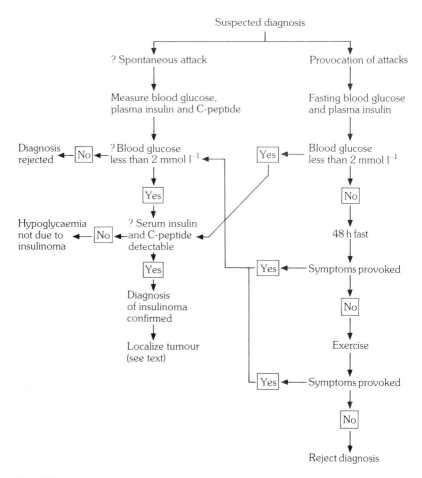

Fig. 5.1 Investigation of fasting hypoglycaemia in adults.

ENDOCRINOLOGY

Thyroid disorders

Clinical features

The clinical spectrum of thyroid disease includes hyperthyroidism, hypothyroidism and goitre.

Hyperthyroidism

This condition results from excessive secretion of thyroid hormones (T4 and T3; occasionally T3 alone).

The most important symptoms include nervousness, excessive sweating, heat intolerance and weight loss. The patient may complain of palpitations and breathlessness. There is a tachycardia, tremor, and diffuse enlargement of the thyroid may be evident.

One of the commonest forms is Grave's disease in which the gland is stimulated by an IgG autoantibody. Another antibody is responsible for the eye signs of exophthalmos and ophthalmoplegia which occur in addition to lid retraction (ophthalmic Grave's factor).

Features of thyroid overactivity may not be obvious in the elderly, who simply present with cardiac failure and/or atrial fibrillation. Such patients often have a multi-nodular goitre. Untreated thyrotoxicosis can lead to thyroid crisis, with hyperthermia and cardiac failure and, ultimately, death.

Hypothyroidism

This most commonly occurs due to primary failure of the thyroid gland, rarely due to congenital defect of hormonogenesis, frequently following autoimmune destruction and sometimes after surgical resection or irradiation. Uncommonly, hypothyroidism is secondary to pituitary failure.

The onset is insidious with lethargy, mental slowness and cold intolerance, as well as constipation and menstrual irregularities. There is a dry skin, hoarse voice, puffy face, bradycardia and delay in relaxation of the tendon reflexes.

Goitre

Goitres may be caused by diffuse enlargement, multiple or solitary nodules.

Diffuse goitres accompany Grave's disease and viral thyroiditis (both of which are associated with hyperthyroidism) and hypothyroidism when the gland is then stimulated by thyroid stimulating hormone (TSH).

Multi-nodular goitres are found in the elderly when they sometimes lead to thyrotoxicosis. Single nodules may be functioning (also leading to thyrotoxicosis) or non-functioning. A minority of the latter are malignant, when cervical lymphadenopathy may be evident.

Investigations

The investigations are listed in Table 5.6. It is important to recognize that many patients with classical clinical features can have their diagnosis confirmed with a single blood test.

Table 5.6 Investigation of thyroid disease

Biochemistry	Thyroxine (T4)
	Tri-iodothyronine (T3)
	Thyroid stimulating hormone
	Thyrotrophin releasing hormone test
Immunology	Thyroid antibodies
	Thyroid stimulating immunoglobulin
Radioisotope studies	Scanning: thyroid gland and metastases
	Thyroid uptake studies
Ultrasound	Single non-functioning nodule
Biopsy/Fine needle aspiration	Single non-functioning nodule

Biochemistry

Biochemical tests of thyroid function include serum total thyroxine (T4), total tri-iodothyronine (T3) and TSH estimations.

Typically, thyrotoxic patients will have elevated T4 (and/or T3) and suppressed TSH. Patients with primary hypothyroidism will have depressed T4 and elevated TSH values. The TSH will also be low in those with secondary hypothyroidism.

Occasional difficulties in interpretation are encountered due to changes in the serum-binding protein and other factors. Causes of elevated and reduced levels of T4 are summarized in Tables 5.7 and 5.8.

Some laboratories estimate free T4; this overcomes the problem of changes in the serum-binding protein. Other laboratories use an estimated thyroid-binding protein to derive a free thyroxine index.

Where doubt remains about thyroid status, measuring the TSH response to injected thyrotrophin releasing hormone (TRH) can be helpful, as summarized in Table 5.9. TRH fails to stimulate TSH secretion in the hyperthyroid or euthyroid patient with autonomous secretion.

Immunology

Thyroid antibodies

Titres of greater than 1 in 32 for microsomal antibodies and greater than 1 in 100 for thyroglobulin antibodies indicate significant autoimmune thyroiditis.

Thyroid-stimulating immunoglobulin

Positive receptor assay for thyroid-stimulating immunoglobulins supports a diagnosis of Grave's disease.

Table 5.7 Causes of elevated serum total thyroxine

Hyperthyroidism	
Increased serum-binding protein	
Increased thyroxine binding globulin (TBG)	Inerited TBG excess
	Endogenous oestrogen effect (pregnancy)
	Non-thyroidal causes (liver disease, porphyria, hydatidiform mole)
Increased albumin and thyroxine-binding proalbumin binding (TBPA)	Familial dysalbuminaemic hyperthyroxaemia
	Inherited TBPA excess
Transient hyperthyroxinaemic states	Acute medical illness
	Acute psychiatric illness
	Vomiting of pregnancy
Drugs	Amphetamines
	Amiodarone
	Iodinated contrast medium
	Thyroxine
Peripheral tissue resistance to thyroid hormones	

Table 5.8 Causes of low serum total thyroxine

Hypothyroidism	
Decreased serum-binding protein	
Decreased TBG production	Inherited TBG deficiency
	Chronic liver disease
Excessive TBG loss	Nephrotic syndrome
	Protein-losing enteropathy
Systemic illness	
Drugs	Androgens
	Glucocorticoids
Inhibition of T4 protein binding	
Systemic illness	
Drugs	Salicylates
	Phenytoin
	Fenclofenac
Exogenous T3 therapy	

Radioisotope studies

Scanning with iodine-131 or technetium-99m has been used as a dynamic test of thyroid function for the diagnosis of hyperthyroidism when there is a greater uptake of isotope. However, scans are rarely used for this purpose now.

Scans are required for the evaluation of the extent of retrosternal goitres, localization of ectopic thyroid tissue and establishment of the functional activity of thyroid nodules.

Cold nodules require exploration by ultrasound and aspiration cytology or biopsy.

Diagnostic approach

The diagnostic approaches to patients with suspected hyperthyroidism, hypothyroidism and nodular goitre are summarized in Figs 5.2, 5.3 & 5.4.

Table 5.9 Causes of impaired TSH response to exogenously administered TRH

Increased thyroid hormone feedback
   Hyperthyroidism
   Autonomously functioning thyroid tissue without hyperthyroidism

Impaired pituitary or hypothalmic function
   Pituitary hypothyroidism
   Cushing's syndrome
   Acromegaly
   Depression
   Systemic illness

Drugs
   Glucocorticoids
   Dopamine

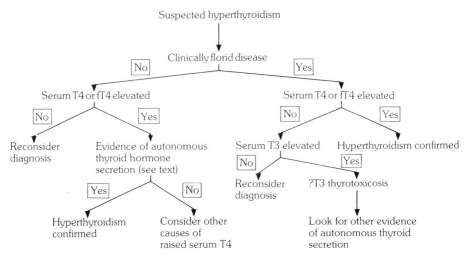

Fig. 5.2 Investigation of suspected hyperthyroidism.

Diseases of the hypothalamus and pituitary gland

Clinical features

Pituitary tumours can cause symptoms in three ways:

1 Secretion of a hormone; examples include growth hormone (acromegaly), adrenocorticotrophic hormone—ACTH (Cushing's disease) and prolactin. A prolactinoma is the commonest secreting tumour.

2 Destruction of surrounding pituitary gland leading to loss of hormone synthesis. Under these circumstances, follicle-stimulating hormone (FSH), luteinizing hormone (LH) and TSH are often the first to be affected. Ultimately, the posterior pituitary and hypothalamus may be damaged causing diabetes insipidus which is characterized by thirst and polyuria.

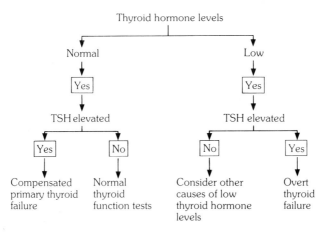

Fig. 5.3 Investigation of hypothroidism.

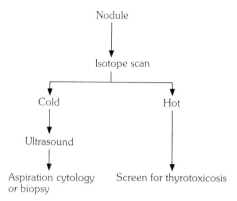

Fig. 5.4 Investigation of thyroid nodule.

3 Invasion of the surrounding structures leading to headaches, cranial nerve palsies and visual field defects, particularly bitemporal hemianopia.

Investigations

Investigations are designed to:
1 Identify a secreted hormone.
2 Assess the residual pituitary function.
3 Look for surrounding structural damage.

Hormone secretion

Serum prolactin is measured. Prolactin is frequently elevated for a variety of reasons, including stress, but high values are often indicative of a pituitary tumour.

In acromegalic patients, growth hormone secretion is high. Single values are difficult to interpret but the failure to suppress growth hormone secretion after a glucose load is characteristic.

Cushing's disease and syndrome are investigated as outlined in Fig. 5.5.

Pituitary function tests

A TRH test and, in the pre-menopausal woman, a luteinizing hormone releasing hormone (LHRH) test, or, in the post-menopausal patient, LH and FSH, gives an indication of residual pituitary function. With prolonged deficiency of ACTH the short synacthen test will also give an impaired response.

An insulin stress test, in which insulin is used to induce hypoglycaemia as a stimulus for ACTH secretion, tests the pituitary–adrenal axis, as assessed by the subsequent measurement of serum cortisol values. However, this procedure is potentially hazardous; it should not be used in patients with ischaemic heart disease and is pointless in the patient with an obvious tumour in whom there is evidence of pituitary insufficiency from the other tests.

In patients with hypothalamic or posterior pituitary damage, diabetes insipidus is suggested by the symptoms of polyuria and thirst; it is distinguished from psychogenic poldipsia by a water deprivation test in which urinary and

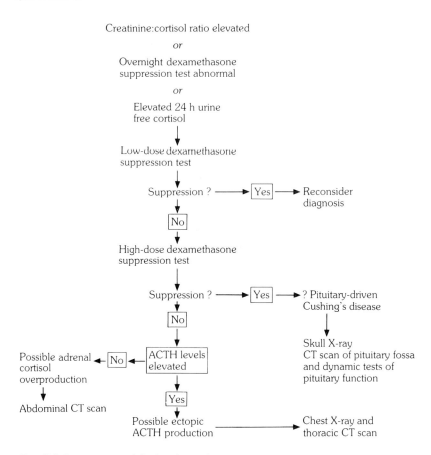

Fig. 5.5 Investigation of Cushing's syndrome.

plasma osmolalities are measured during a prolonged fast. After a defined time the patient receives deamino-D-arginine vasopressin (DDAVP) and the effect on urine volume and osmolality are assessed. However, the test should be terminated if the patient loses 4% of the initial body weight during the investigation. Interpretation of the water deprivation test is demonstrated in Table 5.10.

Table 5.10 Results of fluid deprivation tests

Post-dehydration osmolality		Post-DDAVP osmolality	
Plasma	Urine	Urine	Diagnosis
280–295	750	750	Normal
295	300	300	Nephrogenic diabetes insipidus
295	300	750	Cranial diabetes insipidus
295	300–750	750	? adequate test ? primary polydipsia ? partial cranial diabetes insipidus

Tests of structure

Patients should be examined by a lateral skull X-ray, CT scan of the pituitary fossa and perimetry of the visual fields.

Disease of the adrenal gland

Clinical features

Cushing's syndrome may arise from three separate mechanisms:

1 pituitary overproduction of ACTH (Cushing's disease);

2 autonomous adrenocortical cortisol production (adenoma or carcinoma); and

3 ectopic production of ACTH (e.g. by bronchogenic carcinoma).

The features of truncal obesity, hirsutism, diabetes, osteoporosis and psychiatric disorders are well known.

The adrenal may secrete excessive amounts of aldosterone from either hyperplasia or an adenoma leading to hypertension (Conn's syndrome). These patients can develop symptoms because of the associated hypokalaemia. Phaechromocytoma is another secretory tumour which tends to arise from the adrenal medulla. Apart from hypertension, which is not always intermittent, such patients may experience other symptoms including sweating, palpitations and sensations of impending doom.

Adrenal hypofunction may be autoimmune in origin, when there is often other associated autoimmune disease and adrenal antibodies. Other causes include destruction by tumour, amyloid or tuberculosis. Patients with adrenal insufficiency complain of lassitude, cramps and diarrhoea; pigmentation may be evident due to unsuppressed ACTH secretion. Intercurrent infection or surgical stress may lead to an adrenal crisis with severe hypotension and hyperkalaemia.

Investigations

The investigations undertaken for the diagnosis of Cushing's syndrome are outlined in Fig. 5.5. Table 5.11 summarizes the tests used to establish the cause of Cushing's syndrome.

Figure 5.6 summarizes the steps taken to establish a diagnosis of Conn's syndrome. Tumour localization is by CT scanning of the adrenal glands and also isotope scanning using iodocholesterol.

The diagnosis of phaeochromocytoma is traditionally established by measuring the 24 hour urinary excretion of hydroxymethymandelic acid (HMMA or VMA). Recently, the measurement of plasma catecholamines has been advocated for this purpose. Localization of any suspected tumour is by CT and isotope scanning, the latter with $[^{131}I]$iodobenzyl guanidine (mIBG).

The diagnosis of adrenal failure is outlined in Fig. 5.7.

Diseases of the parathyroid glands

The parathyroid glands secrete parathormone (PTH) which serves to maintain serum calcium through its action on bone resorption and vitamin D metabolism.

Table 5.11 Tests to establish the cause of Cushing's syndrome

Test	Pituitary driven Cushing's	Ectopic ACTH	Adrenal adenoma	Adrenal carcinoma
Diurnal variation plasma cortisol	Absent	Absent	Absent	Absent
Low-dose dexamethasone suppression	Absent	Absent	Absent	Absent
High-dose dexamethasone suppression	Usually present	Usually absent	Absent	Absent
Response to insulin hypoglycaemia	Absent	Absent	Absent	Absent
Metyrapone	Exaggerated	Usually absent	Absent	Absent
Plasma ACTH	Detectable or high	Usually very high	Undetectable	Absent
Other tests	—	—	—	Elevated urinary oxosteroids

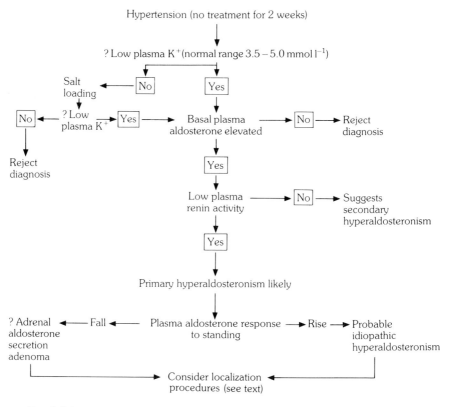

Fig. 5.6 Investigation of hyperaldosteronism.

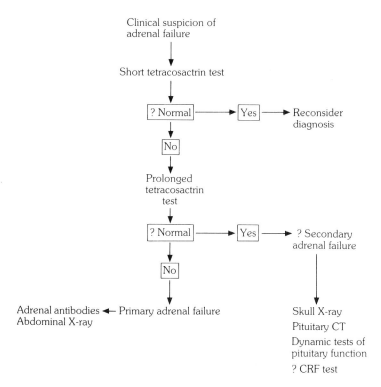

Fig. 5.7 Diagnosis of adrenal failure.

Hyperparathyroidism is relatively common and is one cause of hypercalcaemia. It is caused by an adenoma and is frequently detected during routine blood screening. The investigation of hyperparathyroidism is illustrated in Fig. 5.8.

Hypoparathyroidism causes hypocalcaemia and leads to muscle cramps; it usually follows inadvertent surgical removal. It is rare.

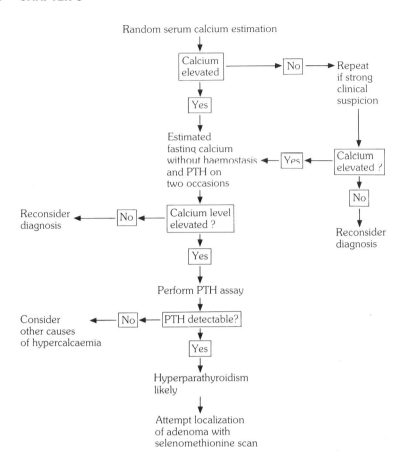

Fig. 5.8 Investigation of hyperparathyroidism.

Chapter 6
Neurology and Psychiatry

Introduction

A careful history and examination is paramount for the assessment of neurological disorders and for choosing appropriate investigations. Specialized investigations are very important for the diagnosis and management of some neurological disorders, e.g. epilepsy, cerebral tumours, subdural haematoma and polymyositis, but are relatively unimportant for others, e.g. migraine, tension headache and Parkinson's disease.

Neurological investigations have evolved rapidly in recent years. Some have revolutionized the management of important neurological disorders, e.g. CT scan, while others are interesting research tools used in a few centres only, e.g. positron emission tomographic (PET) scanning. In the following discussion each of the main techniques will be described briefly; the uses and limitations will be outlined together with rationale for selection of tests.

General symptoms

Symptoms of neurological disease may reflect a primary disorder of the nervous system such as epilepsy, or involvement of the nervous system in a systemic disease process such as vasculitis or secondary carcinoma. Some common neurological presentations are summarized in Table 6.1.

Headache

The commonest causes are migraine and tension headaches, diagnosed on clinical gounds and usually not requiring special investigations. Many patients fear that their new headache indicates tumour; early morning headaches, increasing with coughing, bending, etc. suggest raised intracranial pressure which requires investigation. There are usually additional neurological symptoms. Cranial arteritis must also be considered in the elderly, especially as there is a risk of blindness, if untreated; the erythrocyte sedimentation rate (ESR) is usually, but not invariably, elevated.

Table 6.1 Common neurological presentations

Headache
Epilepsy
Coma or confusional states
Parkinson's disease and other movement disorders
Dementia
Lateralized neurological symptoms
Neuropathies: localized or generalized
Radiculopathy and myelopathies
Muscle disorders
Psychiatric disorders

Epilepsy

Partial or generalized seizures may be clearly described by the patient or a witness. Generalized seizures include absence attacks (petit mal), myoclonus and tonic–clonic (grand mal) seizures. Partial seizures arise from a localized cerebral lesion with retained consciousness (simple) or loss of consciousness (complex). They may spread to become secondary generalized convulsions. Accurate diagnosis is essential to firmly establish the diagnosis, to identify the underlying lesion if possible, to permit discussion of prognosis and to select the appropriate treatment.

Coma or confusion states

Careful assessment of metabolic disorder (e.g. diabetes), drug intoxication, meningitis/encephalitis, stroke, post-ictal confusion and non-convulsive status epilepticus should be considered. Ventilation, BP and pulse rate also need frequent assessment.

Parkinson's disease

Parkinson's disease is recognized from clinical features of tremor, rigidity and hypokinesis. Investigation is usually unnecessary.

Dementia

Dementia presents with impairment of memory and other higher mental functions. Loss of initiative and drive, emotional lability and antisocial behaviour may occur early but are often later features. Dementia is often the result of Alzheimer's disease or multi-infarct dementia. Other conditions such as frontal meningioma, hydrocephalus, subdural haematoma, neurosyphilis and thiamine deficiency should be excluded, as these may be treatable.

Laterialized neurological symptoms

Lateralized neurological disorders such as hemiparesis, hemianopia, hemisensory disorder and dysphasia often arise from stroke but may be caused by tumour or abscess. Multiple sclerosis also causes a wide variety of localized symptoms and signs.

Neuropathies

If sensory and/or motor features are reported distally in the limbs, a generalized peripheral neuropathy is likely. Mononeuropathy, commonly from nerve entrapment, presents with localized numbness, tingling, weakness and wasting.

Radiculopathy and myelopathies

Spondylosis is the commonest cause of localized pain, paraesthesiae and/or weakness. Spasticity, weakness and extensor plantar responses may arise from a compressive cord lesion requiring urgent surgery, from demyelination, or spinal ischaemia.

Myopathies

Myopathies present with weakness and/or muscle pain. Detailed investigation may be needed to establish whether it is a genetically determined dystrophy, a metabolic myopathy, polymyositis or myasthenia.

Psychiatric symptoms

When patients present with psychiatric symptoms, adequate clinical investigation is necessary because some psychiatric disorders are associated with a high risk of physical illness, e.g. alcoholism and drug abuse. Conversely, systemic disease may present with psychiatric symptoms, e.g. thyrotoxicosis with anxiety hypothyroidism with depression. Serological tests for syphilis are no longer justifiable in the absence of clinical indications.

Specific investigations

Electroencephalography (EEG)

Standard EEG recording

The EEG is a record of the low amplitude electrical activity generated by the brain. It is recorded from the scalp, except for highly specialized intracerebral or sphenoidal recordings used in the investigation of some epilepsies.

The recorded potential changes are a summation of complex rhythmical activity of the brain. The main rhythms are:

1 alpha rhythms, at 8–13 Hz, the dominant activity arising posteriorly in the brain, with the eyes closed;

2 beta rhythms, at more than 13 Hz, the fast activity, especially prominent anteriorly;

3 theta activity, at 4–7 Hz; and

4 delta activity, the slowest rhythms at less than 4 Hz.

Additional normal features are lambda waves seen posteriorly and mu (μ) activity at 10–12 Hz, which may be blocked by voluntary movements on the contra-lateral side of the body. In children, the slower rhythms are normally more prominent and recede with 'maturation'. Marked changes occur during sleep, for the alpha rhythms are replaced by slower rhythms at the theta and delta frequencies. Brief high voltage slow waves occur, usually in response to sensory stimuli. Sleep spindles, runs of 12–14 Hz activity, are found by recording from over the central regions. Rapid eye movements (REM) occur in light sleep and are associated with dreaming. Some patients with narcolepsy develop REM sleep within minutes of falling asleep.

Standard EEG recordings are done with eyes open, eyes closed, during hyperventilation to enhance abnormalities and with photic stimulation to see if repetitive flashes induce paroxysmal disturbances.

Artefacts may be physiological, e.g. tremor, pulse, sweating, movement, or they may be electrical artefacts, e.g. interference from nearby electrical equipment or recorder failure. Asymmetries may be induced by craniotomy, removal of an eye, or scalp trauma.

Uses

The EEG is most useful for demonstrating physiological dysfunction in epilepsy and metabolic disorders, but is not valuable for structural disorders, e.g. tumours or hydrocephalus in which the anatomy is shown by CT scan or magnetic resonance imaging (MRI) scan.

Epilepsy

EEG abnormalities which may be found in epilepsy are as follows.

Spike and wave

These are the generalized large amplitude discharges at 3–4 Hz that are characteristic of absence attacks (petit mal) (Fig. 6.1a). They may be precipitated by hyperventilation.

Spike discharges

These are often focal, arising from an area of localized cortical damage (Fig. 6.1b), and are useful in localizing the focal abnormality in patients with partial seizures. As the standard EEG recording does not record from the orbital surface of the frontal lobe or the medial aspects of the temporal lobes, the absence of spikes in a standard recording does not exclude partial seizures.

Spike discharges may also occur bilaterally at the onset of tonic–clonic (grand mal) seizures.

Sharp and slow waves

These also occur with focal abnormalities or bilaterally in patients with partial or generalized seizures. They are less specific for epilepsy than spike discharges for they may be found in people with histories of head injury, migraine and previous ischaemic or inflammatory damage, and even in normal subjects.

Photoconvulsive discharges

These occur with flash frequencies commonly between 14 and 20 Hz but also at other frequencies; they are most prominent in children. More complex patterns of stimulation, e.g. vertical lines, may occasionally elicit discharges.

Slow wave discharges

These may occur in epilepsy and may be rhythmical paroxysms in the delta or theta frequencies.

Fast rhythms

These rarely arise from a focal abnormality and are more commonly from benzodiazepines.

Special techniques for epilepsy

Sleep recording

As paroxysmal features sometimes emerge during sleep, EEG recordings during sleep are used in selected cases where there is a probability of epilepsy despite normal or non-specific standard EEG reports.

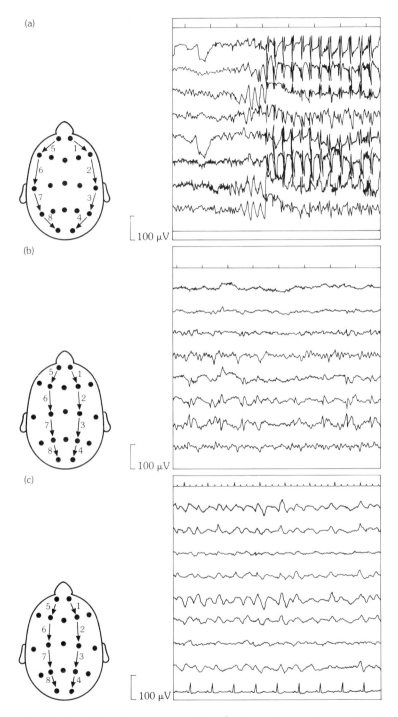

Fig. 6.1 Some EEG abnormalities: (a) $3 \, s^{-1}$ spike and wave discharge in all areas, associated with absence seizures; (b) focal spikes, a focal discharge arising in the left temporal lobe, associated with partial seizures; (c) generalized slow wave abnormality from hepatic encephalopathy. Similar abnormalities occur with other encephalopathies.

Depth recording
Sphenoidal, subdural and/or intracerebral depth recordings are used in specialized laboratories to identify the site of a discharging focus in the work-up for
surgery for partial seizures.

Ambulatory EEG monitoring
This may be used in patients with blackouts of uncertain origin to try to separate
seizures from pseudo-seizures and from cardiac arrhythmias, and to record the
number and duration of spike and wave discharges in patients with absence
attacks. Many centres use ambulatory *tape recording* with 4 or 8 EEG channels.
Simultaneous *EEG and video recording* permit the clinical features to be reliably
recorded together with the EEG.

Limitation of EEG in the study of epilepsy
The interictal EEG may be normal in a patient with epilepsy, and a standard EEG
may be normal during partial seizures from a deep focus.

Conversely, paroxysmal EEG activity is not diagnostic of epilepsy because
episodic discharges may be found in subjects that have never had seizures and
in patients with epilepsy in remission. The EEG recording is not a reliable
method of measuring the response to treatment except for absence seizures. If,
however, the seizures are worsening, further investigations including a repeat
EEG and CT scan may be indicated for the question of whether there is an
expanding lesion, e.g. glioma, underlying the refractory seizures.

Encephalopathies

Metabolic disorders
Increased fast activity may occur with some drugs, most commonly benzodiazepines. Therefore, it is important to give full drug information, including
hypnotics, when requesting EEGs.

The commonest abnormality in metabolic disorders, drug intoxications,
severe electrolyte disturbance or endocrine disorders is slowing of the alpha
activity and/or replacement by theta and delta activity. The EEG has been used
as a measure of hepatic encephalopathy with slowing occurring as the patient
deteriorates and vice versa (Fig.6.1c).

Encephalitis
Slow rhythms, either generalized or focal, the periodic occurrence of large
amplitude complexes, and sometimes superimposed paroxysmal discharges,
may occur. These abnormalities are not specific for encephalitis for they may be
found in other severe brain damage, e.g. severe anoxic or hypoglycaemic brain
damage. In herpes simplex encephalitis the abnormalities are usually severe and
maximal in the frontal and temporal regions.

Degenerative disorders
A low amplitude EEG with prominent fast activity frequently occurs early in
Huntington's chorea. Periodic complexes occur in Creutzfeldt–Jakob disease as

well as in other severe encephalopathies. Mild slowing may occur in early Alzheimer's disease. The EEG is normal in Parkinson's disease unless accompanied by dementia.

Evoked potentials

The visual evoked potential (VEP) is an averaged cortical response to a visual stimulus (either flash stimuli or a checkerboard pattern). The most useful parameter is the latency of a positive occipital cortical potential, usually about 100 ms, the P100. The amplitude of the VEP is more difficult to quantitate reliably. Delay in P100 may occur in optic neuritis, optic nerve compression from tumour, vitamin B_{12} deficiency and inflammatory diseases, such as sarcoidosis.

Uses

The commonest use is for investigating patients with possible multiple sclerosis (MS). In established MS about 90% of patients have delay in the VEPs, but the proportion with abnormalities is lower in patients with possible or probable MS when a reliable diagnosis would be most useful. Commonly the VEPs are delayed in patients with MS without visual symptoms and, if delayed they rarely improve.

Limitations

Abnormal VEPs do not indicate the underlying pathology. As cooperation from the patient is essential for fixating the central spot in the checkerboard, the confused, uncooperative patient is unsuitable except when using the less satisfactory flash stimulus. Adequate visual acuity is essential for fixing; amblyopic eyes may produce asymmetry in the VEP.

Brain-stem evoked potential (BSEP)

The BSEPs are a series of potentials arising in the acoustic nerve (wave I), the cochlear and olivary nuclei (waves II and III), the lateral lemniscus (wave IV), the inferior colliculus (wave V) and the subcortical structures (waves VI and VII). They are used in the investigation of acoustic neuromas in some centres and in the identification of brain-stem lesions. Abnormalities may be found in MS but also in other disorders that affect the brain-stem, such as head injury, stroke and tumour.

Somatosensory evoked potentials (SEP)

SEPs are recorded over the spinal cord and the brain in response to peripheral stimulation of the skin. They are sometimes useful in measuring conduction through the brachial or lumbar plexus. The central conduction time from the cord to the cerebral cortex is also measured.

Investigation of neuromuscular disorders

Nerve conduction studies

Peripheral nerve conduction studies are widely used for the investigation of both generalized neuropathies and localized lesions (e.g. entrapment neuropathies).

Table 6.2 Nerve conduction velocities and latencies

Nerve	Conduction velocities range (m s^{-1})		Distal latencies (mean (m s^{-1}) $\pm$SD)	
	Motor	Sensory	Motor	Sensory
Ulnar	47–73	45–60	2.9 ± 0.4	2.9 ± 0.4
Median	47–72	45–60	3.7 ± 0.4	3.4 ± 0.5
Common peroneal	42–67		4.7 ± 0.8	
Posterior tibial	40–67		5.1 ± 1.3	

NB: H-reflex latency (m s^{-1}) 25–34; F-wave latency (upper limb) (m s^{-1}) <30.

Both motor and sensory conduction can be recorded. The normal findings in the most commonly studied nerves are shown in Table 6.2.

These techniques record the rate of conduction in the large, rapidly conducting axons (alpha motor neurone and large sensory fibres) and this is normal provided that some large axons remain intact. Conduction is faster in myelinated fibres than in non-myelinated fibres because of the rapid conduction between the nodes of Ranvier (saltatory conduction). Therefore, diseases which produce demyelination in peripheral nerves, e.g. Guillain-Barré syndrome or diabetes, slow the conduction greatly, often to 20–30 m s^{-1} or less. In contrast, neuropathies that predominantly damage the axons, e.g. most drug-induced neuropathies, may slow conduction velocity only slightly, unless there is profound axonal loss including the largest axons.

The median, ulnar and common peroneal nerves are most easily studied but the posterior tibial and radial conductions may also be measured. The techniques for measuring median conductions are illustrated in Fig. 6.2.

For *motor* conduction, nerves are stimulated at two points and the latencies to the electromyography (EMG) responses or motor action potential (MAP) are recorded. The difference between the latencies from proximal and distal sites of stimulation allows the conduction velocity to be calculated, after estimation of the length of the nerve.

Sensory action potentials (SAP) are much lower amplitude and more difficult to measure than the EMG responses, but the method of calculation of conduction velocities is similar to that used for motor conductions. The amplitude reflects the number of conducting axons and the rate of conduction or dispersion of the potential during conduction. Averaging techniques may be required. The SAP, like the MAP, may be reduced in axonal neuropathies.

F- and H-waves
In F-wave recording the stimulus is applied to a peripheral nerve, usually ulnar or median; conduction occurs retrogradely to the anterior horn cell and then back to a muscle from which an EMG is recorded. The H-wave (first described by Hoffman) is a late EMG response to a peripheral nerve stimulus with conduction via a monosynaptic relay in the spinal cord. Both F- and H-waves were developed to try to measure conduction proximally through brachial or lumbosacral plexuses or the roots.

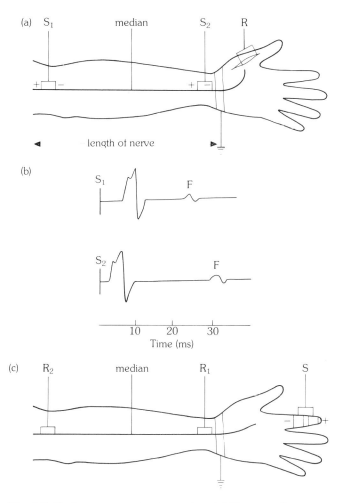

Fig. 6.2 Median nerve conduction studies. (a) Motor conduction: stimuli are applied proximally at S_1 and distally at S_2. The EMG is recorded from opponens pollicis or abductor pollicis brevis (R). (b) The latencies between the stimuli S_1 and S_2 and the EMG responses are measured. The conduction velocity is calculated from the difference in the latencies and the length of the nerve. Note also the late F waves (see text). (c) Sensory conduction, stimulating the skin (S) and recording over the median nerve (R_1 and R_2).

Uses

Entrapment neuropathies and other mononeuropathies
Conduction block from demyelination occurs in mild and moderate nerve entrapment while in severe compression axonal loss with Wallerian degeneration also occurs.

Median. Delay in conduction in the median nerve at the wrist occurs in the carpal tunnel syndrome. This is more sensitively measured by sensory than by motor conduction. A better method is to measure conduction through the compressed segment of the nerve—the wrist–palm latency. These tests are useful and usually reliable. They are difficult to interpret post-operatively as some conduction block often persists. The rare proximal median entrapment at the pronator teres can also be identified.

Ulnar. Conduction may be slowed around the elbow but conduction within the normal range does not exclude mild ulnar nerve entrapment. A distal lesion in the palm also may be shown.

Common peroneal. Slow conduction around the neck of the fibula can be measured.

Posterior tibial. Conduction around the medial malleolus can be measured in patients who may have a tarsal tunnel syndrome.

Generalized neuropathies
Generalized slowing may suggest a demyelinating neuropathy, while reduction of the SAP and MAP is evidence for an axonal neuropathy. Even the Guillain-Barré syndrome, in which there is striking demyelination, may have normal peripheral nerve conduction, except the F-wave latencies, especially in the early stages, because the demyelination is maximal proximally, predominantly in the nerve roots.

Electromyography (EMG)

EMG recordings are made with concentric needle electrodes or with surface recordings. The EMG is used to investigate both neuropathic and myopathic disorders.

Neuropathy
At rest there may be *fibrillation* in which low amplitude (less than 20 μV) short duration potentials arise spontaneously in single denervated muscle fibres (Fig. 6.3a). *Fasciculation* is the spontaneous discharge of a motor unit, and is of larger amplitude (up to 2–4 mV). As fasciculation may be benign, especially with

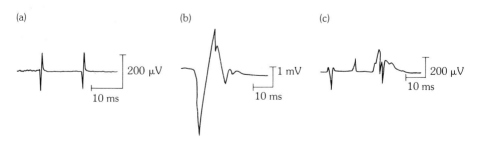

Fig. 6.3 Some EMG abnormalities: (a) fibrillation; (b) high amplitude, long duration potentials, as in motor neurone disease; (c) low amplitude polyphasic potentials as in myopathies.

fatigue, it is not, in itself, diagnostic of a lower motor neurone lesion. *Positive sharp waves* are another feature of denervation. Partial re-innervation of denervated muscle, by sprouting of the remaining nerve terminals, produces abnormally *large, long polyphasic potentials* ('giant potentials') (Fig. 6.3b). On maximal contraction the loss of motor units is seen as gaps in the recruitment of motor units which normally should fill the screen. The activity recorded during maximal contraction is known as the *recruitment* or *interference pattern*.

The EMG is useful for investigating muscle weakness and/or wasting. The diagnosis of a single root level in lumbar or cervical radiculopathies is difficult because of overlap of myotomes. Brachial plexus damage and avulsive root lesions should be studied with EMG and conduction studies. Motor neurone disease may produce widespread denervation including muscles which are not clinically affected; re-innervation with large (giant) motor units may be prominent. Spinal muscular atrophy also produces widespread denervation and the EMG may help to differentiate it from muscular dystrophy. Polyneuropathies may cause diffuse denervation.

The EMG may be helpful after nerve injury. Fibrillation develops after about 10 days. Prominent persistent fibrillation suggests axonal damage. In the early stages of recovery, EMG evidence of voluntary contraction is seen before movement is seen clinically.

Limitations

The EMG cannot differentiate between various types of neuropathies. It is of no value for upper motor neurone lesions except that gapping in the recruitment pattern occurs. Patients need to co-operate both for relaxation, when failure of relaxation may be mistaken for fasciculation, and for maximal contraction when functional weakness may produce apparent gapping of the recruitment pattern. The interpretation of polyphasic potentials, mean amplitudes and durations is subjective and methods of quantitating the EMG are being developed in specialized laboratories.

Myopathies

In myopathies, damage to the muscle fibres which comprise the motor units results in short, small polyphasic (four or more phases) potentials (Fig 6.3c). As the number of motor units is normal (unless the muscle is profoundly affected) the recruitment pattern is full. The specific cause of a myopathy cannot usually be identified except for a few examples. In myotonia high frequency discharges produce a 'dive-bomb' sound on the speaker with insertion of the needle. In polymyositis, fibrillation may occur, and spontaneous activity may occur in rare metabolic myopathy, e.g. acid maltase deficiency.

Additional EMG techniques

Repetitive stimulation

Undue muscle fatigue may be investigated by recording the surface EMG with repetitive supra-maximal stimulation of nerves. In myasthenia gravis there may be a decremental response with repeated stimuli. In the myasthenic syndrome of Eaton–Lambert the EMG response may be facilitated by exercise.

The test has declined in importance in recent years with the development of acetylcholine receptor antibody estimation and single fibre EMG recordings.

Single-fibre EMG
This technique has been introduced into specialist units in recent years. It records the differences in timing in the firing of different fibres within part of a motor unit. Normally there is little scatter or 'jitter' in the timing but in myasthenia gravis the 'jitter' increases. Single fibre recordings may also be used to measure the density of innervation of a motor unit. This 'fibre density' is increased in motor neurone disease but not in demyelinating neuropathies where there is impaired conduction but no re-innervation.

Muscle biopsy

Muscle biopsy is an important tool for investigating some neuromuscular disorders. It can be taken by percutaneous needle biopsy or by an open biopsy under general or local anaesthesia. A muscle should be selected which is mildly or moderately affected because the grossly damaged muscle may be replaced by fat or fibrous tissue. The biopsy should be sent fresh to the laboratory for:

1 histological examination for vascular abnormalities, inflammatory cells and changes in fibre size and shape;

2 histochemical stains for muscle enzymes (e.g. phosphorylase); and

3 electron microscopical (EM) examination, in selected cases, for organelles or other ultrastructural changes, e.g. in congenital myopathies.

The biopsy may show neuropathic or myopathic features. In neuropathies there may be selective loss of muscle fibres innervated by type I or type II fibres (type I contain predominantly oxidative enzymes and have slow, fatigue-resisting twitches, while type II have predominantly glycolytic enzymes with fast twitches that fatigue rapidly). Diagnostic histological changes may be found in the muscular dystrophies. In inflammatory myopathies cellular infiltration, especially around blood vessels and muscle necrosis, may be found. In the inherited metabolic myopathies diagnostic changes may be seen on histochemistry, e.g. phosphorylase deficiency in McArdle's syndrome. In the rare mitochondrial myopathies histological and EM changes occur. Muscle biopsy is indicated in patients with possible myositis to establish a firm basis for treatment. A biopsy may provide a diagnosis in polyarteritis nodosa.

Blood and miscellaneous tests

Creatine kinase (CK)
CK concentrations in the blood increase with muscle necrosis. In normal subjects the concentrations are usually below 100 iu but muscle exertion in some may increase the levels to 200–300 iu. Therefore, a slight increase in a random sample may be due to preceding exertion, and it is wise to repeat the sample after rest.

The concentrations are greatly elevated to several thousand iu after:

1 muscle trauma;
2 inflammatory myopathies, e.g. polymyositis;
3 Duchenne and Becker dystrophies; and
4 acute drug-induced myopathy, e.g. alcoholic myopathy.

Less-marked increases occur with limb–girdle dystrophy. In facioscapulo-humeral dystrophy the CK may be normal. Normal CK may be found in myopathies associated with metabolic bone disease and endocrine disorders. Slight increases may occur in motor neurone disease.

Myoglobinuria

This is additional evidence for massive muscle necrosis and may cause renal failure. Increased CK and myoglobinuria are found in idiopathic paroxysmal myoglobinurias.

Acetylcholine receptor antibodies

These are IgG antibodies to cholinergic receptors in skeletal muscle. The measurement is useful in the diagnosis of myasthenia gravis because it is positive in about 90% of established cases but it cannot be used as an indicator of prognosis or response to treatment.

'Tensilon' test

Edrophonium chloride (Tensilon) is a short-acting anticholinesterase used only for the diagnosis of myasthenia gravis and in patients with established myasthenia with prominent weakness to decide if they are underdosed (i.e. still myasthenic) or overdosed (i.e. cholinergic block). Weak muscles are selected for careful assessment before and after injection. A test dose of 2 mg is given i.v.; wait 1 min for undue sensitivity or allergy and then give the remaining 8 mg. Increased power usually develops within 20–60 s and commonly wears off in 2–3 min. The patient commonly feels sweaty and dizzy. Some doctors routinely give atropine to block the autonomic adverse effects, and atropine should always be available. An ability to provide emergency ventilation is needed when giving Tensilon to potentially overdosed patients as they may worsen.

Cerebrospinal fluid (CSF) examination

The size of the intracranial CSF pathways is seen with CT scanning which clearly shows hydrocephalus, distorted or small ventricles. The rate of CSF production and clearance is not studied in common clinical practice. The CSF pressure is usually measured at lumbar puncture but intracranial pressure monitoring is used in some centres for assessment of hydrocephalus, and for monitoring after severe head injury.

The CSF is usually sampled at lumbar puncture, although it is occasionally taken from the upper cervical level by experienced radiologists, usually when performing a myelogram at that level.

Lumbar puncture (LP)

The important practical points are to use a sterile technique; to have the spine horizontal and flexed as much as possible; to use the smallest diameter needle that is practical, often 20G or 22G; and to measure the pressure before removing CSF samples. Very obese patients, in whom it is impossible to identify the bony landmarks of the spinous processes, may be punctured more easily sitting up and flexed forward.

Headaches after LP occur as a result of continued leakage of CSF from the puncture site into the adjacent extradural space. They occur unpredictably after LP, but are more frequent with larger needles, and may last for a few hours or for more than 10 days. At its worst the headache and vomiting suggest meningitis, but there is clear relief with lying down and worsening with sitting or standing. The patient should remain in bed, and take plenty of fluids. In rare cases with intractable post-LP headache 'patching' may be done with injection of venous blood to the site of leakage.

There is a common tradition that patients should be kept in bed for 24 h to prevent a post-LP headache but a much shorter time such as 2–4 hrs is satisfactory. Therefore, LP can be practised as an out-patient procedure in non-urgent cases.

CSF should be examined for its colour. Minor degrees of *xanthochromia* can be easily missed unless the fluid is compared with water. A yellow colour suggests either blood or a striking increase in the CSF protein. Turbid fluid suggests the presence of cells. The CSF samples should be sent for quantification of total protein, often IgG (or an IgG : albumin ratio), oligoclonal bands and for typing and counting of cells. Request glucose, serology or cytology if indicated. Chloride estimations are not useful.

The traditional Queckenstedt test to show spinal or venous block no longer has a useful place in neurological investigation.

The normal CSF pressure is less than $180 \, mmH_2O$. Slight increases may occur in the tense patient. In patients with possible increased intracranial pressure an LP should not be done, because of the risk of coning, unless there is no evidence for a mass lesion on CT scan or MRI studies. The pressure may be increased to $300–400 \, mmH_2O$ in benign intracranial hypertension.

Indications for LP

The abnormal findings in a variety of conditions are shown in Table 6.3.

The following are comments on the indications for, and limitations of, CSF examinations.

Suspected meningitis

CSF examination is essential to confirm the diagnosis and to obtain an organism in patients with possible bacterial infection. In cases with focal signs and raised intracranial pressure, when abscess is considered, an urgent CT scan (or other investigation) is necessary because an LP may be hazardous. In chronic meningitides such as fungal or tuberculous meningitis, the problem should be discussed with a bacteriologist to encourage the search for the organisms with Indian ink or Ziehl–Nielsen stains, especially in a patient with impaired immunity.

Table 6.3 CSF in neurological disorders

Condition	Total protein (IgG) $(mg\,l^{-1})$	Glucose ratio CSF : blood	Cells*	Other
Normal	400 (55)	0.6	5 L	Pressure $<180\,mmH_2O$
Pyogenic meningitis	800–4000	Often 0	P + + +	Varied organisms pressure ↑
Tuberculous meningitis	800–4000	Low	L <400 P ±	ZN-staining bacteria; clot on standing
Viral meningitis	400–2000	N	L <2000	–
Neurosyphilis	400–2000 ↑	N	L <12	TPHA, FTA, VDRL + †
Multiple sclerosis	400–1000 ↑ (in 1/3)	N	L 5–30	–

* L = lymphocytes; P = polymorphs.
† TPHA = *Treponema pallidum* haemagglutination test; FTA = fluorescent *Treponema* antigen-absorbent test; VDRL = Venereal Disease Research Laboratory.

Subarachnoid haemorrhage
CSF examination is used to confirm the presence of blood in the CSF. This differs from the traumatic 'blood' tap in which the CSF runs clearer of blood as it is removed. The CT scan is an important investigation for subarachnoid haemorrhage and, where facilities exist, should be done before LP, unless there is a strong suspicion of meningitis.

Demyelinating disease
In demyelinating disease, immunoglobulins are produced within the central nervous system (CNS) and enter the CSF. Various methods of expressing the increase in globulins have been described. The IgG : albumin ratio is widely used:

$$\frac{IgG\ in\ CSF}{IgG\ in\ plasma} \times \frac{albumin\ in\ CSF}{albumin\ in\ plasma}\ .$$

The normal ratio is less than 0.7. In addition, oligoclonal bands in CSF may be found in patients with an immunological disorder of the CNS.

These tests are abnormal in about 85% of established cases of MS but they may be normal in early disease when a diagnosis is being sought. Measurements of IgG are not useful as a guide to severity or prognosis of MS.

Increased IgG occurs in a wide variety of other disorders, e.g. neurosyphilis, sarcoidosis, lymphomas, in systemic lupus erythematosus (SLE) of the CNS, Guillain-Barré syndrome and in encephalitis. Dramatic increases in the IgG occur in subacute sclerosing panencephalitis together with increased measles titres in blood and CSF.

Neurosyphilis
Measurement of the IgG has largely replaced the traditional tests using colloidal gold as IgG may be significantly elevated, together with total protein and lymphocytes. Sequential changes may be used to assess the course of treatment. The *Treponema pallidum* haemagglutination (TPHA) test and the fluorescent

Treponema antigen-absorbent (FTA) tests are more specific than the Venereal Disease Research Laboratory (VDRL) test and should be measured in blood as well as in CSF. In late treated neurosyphilis levels may revert to normal.

Neoplastic disease
CSF examination is usually of no value and is potentially hazardous (because of coning) in the investigation of patients with possible tumours of the brain. Nevertheless, cytological examination for malignant cells in patients with possible meningeal metastases, e.g. adenocarcinoma, or with reticuloses may be useful in confirming a diagnosis. Here CT scanning should precede LP to exclude a mass lesion. The protein may be elevated but, except in very active carcinomatous meningitis, the glucose is not decreased.

Guillain-Barré Syndrome
In infective polyneuritis the CSF protein increases but the cells remain normal. This increase may evolve gradually over the first 3 weeks, plateau for several weeks and then gradually return to normal. Thus the CSF protein in the first few days of the illness may be normal. Striking elevation may occur with levels over 2 g l^{-1}, at which level the CSF may have a xanthochromic appearance. The IgG may be elevated.

Miscellaneous inflammatory disease
Increased protein, cells and IgG may occur in sarcoidosis and Behçet's syndrome.

Contra-indications to LP
These include the following.
1 Increased intracranial pressure of uncertain cause, with focal signs, headache, nausea, vomiting or papilloedema. The absence of papilloedema does not exclude raised pressure. The hazard is coning, which may occur within minutes or hours of the puncture, with a deteriorating neurological state, including dysfunction: coma, changing pulse, respiration, blood pressure, dilating pupils.
2 An acute spinal cord syndrome when a myelogram is the appropriate investigation.
3 Infection at the site of the puncture.
4 Bleeding disorders.

Imaging techniques

Skull and brain

Techniques available

Skull X-rays
These are simple, widely available investigations. The usual views used are lateral, posterio-anterior, Townes (30° fronto-occipital projection) and basal.

Views of the internal auditory canal, coned views of the pituitary fossa, special orbital views, or radiology of the sinuses, are very important for some problems.

CT scans

These use complex computerized analysis of X-rays to give reconstructed views of intracranial structures. They provide useful anatomical information but are not useful in physiological abnormality, e.g. epilepsy and drug effects on the brain.

Magnetic resonance imaging (MRI)

This was previously called nuclear magnetic resonance and uses computation of the displacement of protons in a strong magnetic field to give impressive views of the brain and spinal cord. It is slower than CT scanning but has some advantages. It shows plaques in multiple sclerosis much more accurately than a CT scan and gives better resolution close to bone, e.g. for pituitary tumours. Sagittal sections are very useful for the posterior fossa, the craniocervical junction and longitudinal views of the spinal cord.

Isotope scanning

This has been largely replaced by CT scanning which gives superior anatomical detail. Nevertheless, isotope scanning gives a qualitative view of blood flow and may show moderate or large arteriovenous malformations, subdural haematomas, some tumours and large infarcts.

An important recent development is single photon emission computer tomography (SPECT) which uses an isotope, technetium, attached to a lipophilic molecule, hexamethylene propyleneamine oxime (HMPAO). This crosses the blood brain barrier, enters cerebral cells and there becomes hydrophilic; it is therefore retained for some hours to permit scanning. It reflects the blood flow and metabolism at the time of injection of HMPAO. This has a place in the investigation of patients with focal seizures being considered for surgery as it may show hypermetabolism immediately postictally and hypometabolism interictally.

Another type of isotope scan uses radio-iodine labelled albumin (RISA) introduced into the CSF at an LP. It normally mixes rapidly with CSF and flows up over the brain to be re-absorbed by bulk flow through the arachnoid granulations. It may be used for the investigation of normal pressure hydrocephalus (the re-absorption is grossly delayed to 48–72 h). It may also be used in the search for the site of CSF leaks, e.g. in recurrent meningitis.

Arteriography

The carotid arteries need to be seen in patients that are candidates for carotid endarterectomy. Non-invasive ultrasonic methods may show turbulent or reduced flow from severe or moderate stenosis, a complete block or small ulcerating atheromatous plaques. Carotid arteriography is required, either with direct puncture of the common carotid artery or selective cannulation of the origins of the major arteries in the chest. Digital vascular imaging (DVI) using computer subtraction of bone images gives good definition of the extracranial carotid arteries but the views of intracranial arteries are not good. DVI can be done in an out-patient and all the major arteries are seen after the contrast injection without the need for multiple punctures or cannulations.

Positron emission tomographic (PET) scan
This is a research technique that computes the distribution of radioisotopes in the brain. The images do not have the anatomical detail of CT or MRI scans but reflect metabolic changes. Isotopes of glucose or oxygen give information about cerebral perfusion and oxidative metabolism. There is scope for important new developments using labelled drugs and neurotransmitters.

Cerebral blood flow
Such studies use radioactive xenon given intravenously or by inhalation. The technique yields very sophisticated information on cerebral blood flow but has not yet found a use in clinical practice.

Clinical problems to be studied: indications and limitations

Cranial trauma
Plain skull radiology is widely used in head injuries. In mild head injuries with concussion only, without headache, vomiting or additional neurological features, the indications are often medico-legal only. In more severe trauma X-rays may show simple depressed or compound fractures of the vault or fractures of the base of the skull which are important because of associated brain damage, cranial nerve lesions, injury to blood vessels (e.g. middle meningeal artery) or injury to sinuses (risk of infection). Displacement of a calcified pineal gland indicates a mass lesion and the need for further studies, especially a CT scan.

The CT scan is very important in complicated head injuries. Haemorrhages are very clearly shown, allowing extradural, subdural and intracerebral haematomas to be identified. Occasionally chronic subdural haematomas are difficult to separate from adjacent brain (they become isodense), but, nevertheless, are seen because of a mass effect. Hydrocephalus is easily recognized. Local or diffuse oedema can be seen. Therefore, important management decisions on whether to remove a haematoma, identification of its precise site and the differentiation from non-surgical problems can be made on adequate information. Finally, the longer term problems of severe head injury, e.g. hydrocephalus and cortical atrophy, can be identified.

Gradual onset dementia
Plain skull radiology is relatively unimportant unless it shows local skull erosive or sclerotic changes from a frontal tumour, especially a meningioma.

The CT scan is not always diagnostic. One problem is identifying the limits of normal atrophy on a CT scan in an elderly person because of the wide variation in the size of the cerebral sulci and ventricles in the elderly. The CT scan may be normal in early Alzheimer's disease. The CT scan is also normal in patients with metabolic causes for their mental impairment, e.g. hypothyroidism, drug adverse effects and in degenerative disorders such as Parkinson's disease complicated by dementia. In the very elderly patient with failing mental faculties, a CT scan is unlikely to change the management and therefore may be unnecessary. Nevertheless, a CT scan may show or exclude hydrocephalus in a patient with dementia when accompanied by atypical gait and/or incontinence, especially with a history of previous head injury, subarachnoid haemorrhage or meningitis. It may show multiple areas of atrophy in patients with multi-infarct dementia, frontal or temporal lobe tumours or a subdural haematoma.

In patients with dementia and hydrocephalus it is commonly difficult to know whether the patient will be improved by a shunt or whether the atrophy is too extensive. Both RISA (radio-iodine labelled serum albumin) scanning and intracranial pressure monitoring are used but it is unclear which is more useful.

Focal neurological problems or confusional states
In patients with the recent onset of a neurological problem, such as hemiparesis, dysphasia or hemianopia, a CT scan is more useful than plain skull X-rays. The CT features of a *cerebral infarct* may evolve over 36 h with diminished attenuation, suggestive of oedema, and enhancement with contrast (Fig. 6.4). A mass effect occasionally occurs in large infarcts. There is a gradual improvement in subsequent weeks often to leave a residual area of diminished attenuation reflecting atrophy. In contrast, *haematomas* produce radiodense lesions which usually resolve gradually over weeks or months. A small proportion of patients with haematomas producing progressive neurological deterioration require surgery. Primary and secondary brain *tumours* are usually seen easily but a precise diagnosis demands additional clinical information and a biopsy. Meningiomas usually have distinctive appearances at their sites of predilection in the parasagittal region, the convexity, the olfactory groove, the sphenoid wing, clivus and the cerebellopontine angle (Fig. 6.5). Metastatic tumours tend to be rounded. The gliomas often have irregular margins and some have cavitated centres. All may have surrounding oedema. Slowly growing tumours, e.g. some

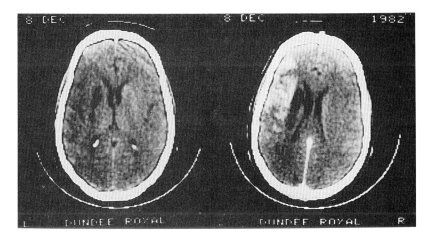

Fig. 6.4 CT scans of a recent left middle cerebral infarct: (left) no contrast; (right) with contrast.

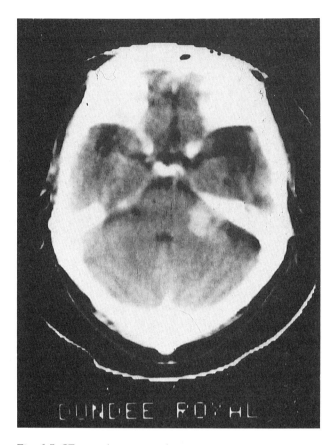

DUNDEE ROYHL

Fig. 6.5 CT scan showing a right acoustic neuroma.

oligodendrogliomas and meningiomas, old abscesses, large aneurysms and vascular malformations may calcify. Cerebral abscesses show prominent abnormalities.

The MRI scan shows tumours clearly, and may show diagnostic features in cerebral infarction and haemorrhage.

In *confusional states* caused by metabolic abnormalities or drugs the CT scan is normal except where there is oedema, e.g. after severe hypoglycaemia. The role of the CT scan is to study the patient without a metabolic explanation for the recent mental impairment, for there may be inflammatory, vascular or malignant disease. In herpes simplex encephalitis areas of diminished attenuation are seen in temporal and frontal regions. Other forms of encephalitis are less distinctive. Areas of diminished attenuation may also occur in vascular disease, including the cerebral complications of SLE. Diminished attenuation in the periventricular regions occurs in severe MS and in cerebrovascular disease.

Subarachnoid haemorrhage
A CT scan may show blood in the ventricular system, and/or a haematoma at the site of the bleed. Radiodense areas may be seen with an arteriovenous

malformation (AVM) and vascular markings are seen on contrast enhancement. Very small AVMs may rarely be missed. Carotid arteriography should be done in patients that are in a satisfactory clinical state after a recent subarachnoid haemorrhage to show the aneurysm or AVM, if present (Fig. 6.6). Skull radiology may show calcification in vascular lesions, e.g. large aneurysm.

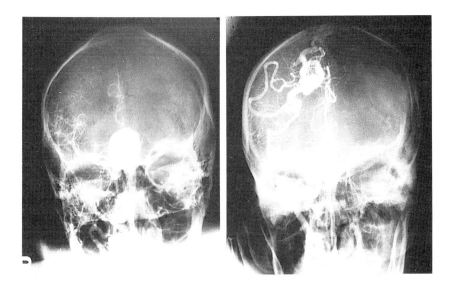

Fig. 6.6 Arteriograms showing: (left) giant cerebral aneurysm; (right) arteriovenous malformation.

Cranial neuropathies
Skull radiology has an important role in investigation of cranial neuropathies because CT scans do not show bone structures satisfactorily. Skull X-rays including orbital views may show the orbit, the superior orbital fissure, the pituitary fossa and the sphenoidal ridge in patients with optic, III, IV, V and VI nerve lesions. The base of skull views help in showing the exit foramina in patients with trigeminal and with X, XI and XII nerve lesions. Internal auditory meati should be examined in patients with deafness, tinnitus or vertigo (?acoustic neuroma), with special views if they are not seen on standard films.

CT scans are important for showing intracranial lesions causing cranial neuropathies, e.g. an inferior frontal tumour compressing the olfactory tract producing anosmia, a pituitary tumour extending upwards to involve the optic chiasm, or a parapituitary tumour or aneurysm compressing the III, IV, V or VI nerves. A large cerebellopontine angle tumour, e.g. acoustic neuroma, may be seen but small tumours within the internal auditory canal are not. These require highly specialized techniques in which the canal is outlined with contrast (internal auditory meatogram).

Spinal imaging

Methods

Spinal X-rays

Anterior-posterior (AP) and lateral views of the spine show the vertebral body, the pedicles, the transverse processes, and the spinous processes. Views in flexion and extension are taken if there is a question of subluxation. AP views through the mouth are taken to show the odontoid peg in patients with trauma. Oblique views show the exit foramina and the facet joints.

Myelography and radiculography

Water soluble contrast is now always used for contrast studies of the spinal canal. It is usually given via LP but can be introduced at a cervical level for better views of the cervical region or to define the upper end of a spinal block. Myelography may show an expanded cord, e.g. syrinx or glioma, or it may show displacement of the cord by an intradural mass, e.g. a neuroma or meningioma (Fig. 6.7), or by extradural disease, e.g. intervertebral discs, or metastatic tumours.

CT scan

The CT scan shows the vertebrae in the surrounding soft tissues and the spinal cord, usually in transverse section. Recent scanners permit sagittal views. Contrast may be introduced to help to define the pathology. CT scanning does not replace myelography.

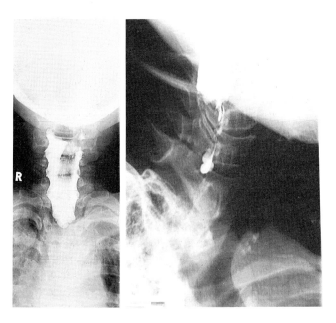

Fig. 6.7 Cervical myelogram showing cord compression at C4 level from neuroma: (left) AP; (right) lateral.

MRI scan
This provides views of the spinal cord especially with sagittal views, and, where available, usually replaces the more invasive procedure of myelography.

Spinal angiography
This is a highly skilled radiological technique occasionally used in the investigation of possible spinal AVMs.

Indications
These problems may present separately or together.

Spinal pain or stiffness
The commonest causes of spinal pain are abnormalities in the soft tissues which do not show on X-ray. As spondylosis is universal in older patients the finding of spondylotic changes on an X-ray must be interpreted together with the clinical features. Degenerative disease at the facet joints also commonly causes pain. Acute pain from vertebral collapse, tumour or trauma may be shown with spinal X-rays. Other diseases of the spine are shown, e.g. ankylosing spondylitis.

Radiculopathy
When patients present with weakness, pain, sensory loss with/without loss of local tendon reflexes, spinal X-rays are indicated. They may show posterior osteophytosis and encroachment upon exit foramina by bone. In the lumbar region the lumbar canal may be narrowed (spinal stenosis). Other changes such as spondylolisthesis are readily seen. If surgery is contemplated or there is still a diagnostic problem myelography, radiculography or MRI is indicated.

Myelopathy
Patients with spinal cord disease need plain radiology and, if the diagnosis is unclear, myelography or spinal MRI. Emergency studies are indicated if the deterioration has been rapid over hours or a few days, for urgent decompression may be needed. A diagnostic LP alone is indicated only if there is strong evidence for a medical, e.g. transverse myelitis, rather than a surgical lesion, e.g. spinal meningioma.

Blood tests and miscellaneous investigations

A variety of blood tests can provide important diagnostic information. A blood count may show evidence of macrocytic anaemia suggestive of vitamin B_{12} deficiency which is sometimes associated with optic atrophy or peripheral neuropathy in addition to the classical syndrome of subacute combined degeneration of the cord. More commonly this finding in patients with neurological symptoms is suggestive of ethanol abuse. Conversely, poly-cythaemia can lead to cerebrovascular disease. A very high erythrocyte sedimentation rate (ESR) raises the possibility of vasculitis which presents to the neurologist in various ways, including mononeuritis multiplex, headache or stroke.

Abnormalities of the liver function tests may suggest alcohol abuse (macrocytosis of the blood film enhances such suspicion) or malignancy. Hypokalaemia, thyroid abnormalities and low vitamin D status may be found in patients who complain of muscle weakness. Patients who are suffering from epileptic fits should have glucose and calcium concentrations measured. The estimation of blood ethanol can be useful in those who will not admit to drinking in spite of strong clinical suspicion.

Serology will confirm the presence of viral infection in patients with meningitis or encephalitis (e.g. mumps, herpes simplex, AIDS) and in some cases of vasculitis, e.g. with the hepatitis B virus. Serology is also used to establish a diagnosis of neurosyphilis, now rare.

The use of muscle enzymes (CK) and acetylcholine receptor antibodies in the investigation of neuromuscular disorders has already been discussed.

Serum anticonvulsant levels in the management of epilepsy

1 Anticonvulsant serum levels are to be used as an approximate guide to anticonvulsant dosage only, for both the upper and the lower limits are not clearly defined; e.g. a patient may have seizures controlled with serum levels beneath the range, or may have no adverse effects above the range.

2 Serum levels are useful in:

(a) patients with continued seizures, i.e. is he/she refractory to the drug(s) with adequate serum levels or is there either an inadequate dose or non-compliance?; and

(b) patients with adverse effects, e.g. can drowsiness be attributed to high serum levels?

The measurements are especially useful in patients with polytherapy where drug interactions may occur, e.g. valproate increases phenobarbitone levels; phenobarbitone may increase/decrease or not affect phenytoin levels.

3 The value of serum levels of valproate as a guide to therapy is not established.

4 Phenytoin has saturable kinetics, i.e. serum levels may rise rapidly within and above the therapeutic range with small dose increments.

5 There is no need to regularly monitor serum levels in patients with well-controlled epilepsy without adverse effects.

6 Therapeutic ranges:

Phenytoin	$40\text{--}80\ \mu\text{mol l}^{-1}$	$(20\text{--}40\ \mu\text{g ml}^{-1})$
Carbamazepine	$24\text{--}42\ \mu\text{mol l}^{-1}$	$(\ 6\text{--}10\ \mu\text{g ml}^{-1})$
Phenobarbitone	$80\text{--}160\ \mu\text{mol l}^{-1}$	$(20\text{--}40\ \mu\text{g ml}^{-1})$
Valproate	$300\text{--}600\ \mu\text{mol l}^{-1}$	$(50\text{--}100\ \mu\text{g ml}^{-1})$

No range for vigabatrin or benzodiazepines.

7 Timing of blood sample after change of dose: estimate serum levels after 4–5 days or more for phenytoin, 3–4 days for carbamazepine; 3 weeks for phenobarbitone; and 3–4 days for valproate (the times required to reach a new plateau level).

8 Timing of blood samples in relation to dose is not important for phenobarbitone and phenytoin because of long half-lives of the drug; it is more important for carbamazepine in which the half-life is 8–19 h. Ideal times for monitoring efficacy might be a trough and a 5-hour level, but, in practice, sampling usually is determined by the time of the review consultation. Acute toxic dose-related effects (ataxia, diplopia, blurred vision and drowsiness) may occur within 1–2 h and serum level measurement is then reasonable, if there is doubt about the cause of the symptoms.

Chest X-ray

A chest X-ray should be requested in older patients who present with focal signs or peripheral neuropathy, particularly if there is a history of heavy cigarette smoking, when metastatic disease or a non-metastatic syndrome can be responsible for the neurological symptoms.

Carotid ultrasound

Duplex scanning now permits images of the bifurcation of the common carotid into the internal and external carotid arteries, and Doppler techniques estimate flow. This has an important role as a non-invasive study in patients with transient ischaemic attacks (TIA) or small strokes, in whom carotid surgery may be considered. Thus patients with normal carotid arteries may avoid arteriography.

Diagnostic approach for the investigation of common neurological and psychiatric disorders

Headache

1   Is it migraine or tension headache?
2   Are there features of raised intracranial pressure or additional neurological signs?—CT scan.
3   Is cranial arteritis likely?—ESR and arterial biopsy.

Epilepsy

Is it epilepsy?
1   History from patients and witnesses.
2   Carry out EEG; if normal, and diagnostic doubt remains perform sleep EEG; if frequent episodes, video-EEG or ambulatory EEG monitoring.
3   ECG and ECG tape recordings, if possible arrhythmia.
4   Glucose, if possible hypoglycaemia.
5   Carotid ultrasound studies, if possible TIAs.
What is the cause of the seizures?
1   Is there a structural lesion? CT scan in adults with recent seizures, and patients with focal, non-benign EEG abnormalities (MRI, if available).
2   Is there a metabolic cause? Sodium, potassium, calcium, glucose, liver function tests (many patients have no recognizable structural or metabolic cause).

Multiple sclerosis

1   Are there multiple lesions within the CNS? The clinical features are most important. If diagnosis is uncertain, perform MRI scan, if available, or evoked potentials.

2 Is there evidence for immunoglobulin production within the CNS? Perform LP and CSF IgG estimation (also examine for cells and total protein).
3 Is there evidence for an alternative diagnosis? For example,
(a) is there a single compressive lesion of the spinal cord? Perform myelogram or MRI scan.
(b) is there another intracranial lesion? Perform CT scan or MRI scan.
(c) is there an inflammatory or infective disorder such as SLE, or other vasculopathy, sarcoidosis or AIDS? Carry out appropriate investigations.

Neuromuscular disorders

1 Is there a mononeuropathy (usually an entrapment neuropathy)? Carry out nerve conduction studies: EMG, if unclear.
2 Is there a condition predisposing to entrapment neuropathy or mononeuropathy? Glucose, T4, rheumatoid factor (RF), X-rays, only if there is a possible local bone lesion on clinical criteria, e.g. RA wrist.
3 Is there an axonal or demyelinating generalized neuropathy? Perform nerve conduction studies.
4 What is the cause of the generalized neuropathy? Carry out FBC, ESR, T4, B_{12}, folate, glucose, urea and creatinine, LFTs, plasma protein electrophoresis, antinuclear factor (ANF), RF, chest X-ray and other investigations for malignancy—all according to clinical suspicion. Porphyrins and lead levels should be monitored for predominantly motor neuropathies. In acute neuropathy, perform LP for protein and cells.
5 Is there a radiculopathy? Carry out spinal X-rays. Also obtain myelogram, radiculogram and/or CT scan if diagnosis is still uncertain and surgery may be considered. EMG is sometimes helpful.
6 Is there myasthenia gravis? Carry out Tensilon test and acetylcholine receptor antibodies; repetitive EMG recordings and single fibre EMG, if diagnosis still unclear and facilities are available.

Chest X-ray and/or thoracic CT scan for possible thymoma in confirmed myasthenia.

For possible Eaton–Lambert syndrome carry out chest X-ray (?bronchogenic carcinoma) and ESR, ANF, etc. for connective tissue disorder.
7 Is there a myopathy and what is its cause? Carry out EMG, serum CK, muscle biopsy. Additional investigations depend on clinical suspicion:
(a) Endocrine disorder? Perform assays for T4, cortisols or growth hormone.
(b) Polymyositis? Investigate for connective tissue disorder (FBC, ESR, ANF, RF, double stranded DNA (ds DNA)) or for malignancy (chest X-ray, with other investigations according to clinical features).
(c) Muscular dystrophy? Obtain ECG (cardiomyopathy is common).
(d) Other metabolic myopathy? Monitor electrolytes (especially potassium, calcium, phosphate, alkaline phosphatase and LFTs).

Acute confusional state

Despite the difficulties of managing a disturbed, perplexed, elderly patient in the general hospital setting, facilities for accurate clinical diagnosis are essential for instituting appropriate treatment.

1 Is there primary intracranial disease? Carry out CT scan, EEG, CSF.

2 Is there an acute metabolic disorder? Monitor urea and creatinine, electrolytes, LFTs, T4, vitamin B_{12}, folate, blood glucose, calcium and phosphate (rarely magnesium); carry out drug assay (phenytoin, barbiturate, lithium, thiamine—if available), chest X-ray (?tumour, cardiac failure) and monitor blood gases in chronic obstructive airways disease (?hypoxia).

3 Is this non-convulsive status epilepticus? Obtain EEG.

4 Urine microscopy and culture.

Dementias

The dementias are commonly related to degenerative conditions such as Alzheimer's disease or vascular conditions, e.g. multi-infarct dementia. Totally reversible dementias are rare.

1 Is there a reversible metabolic disorder? Carry out T4, urea and creatinine, electrolytes, drug assays (for chronic toxicity), LFTs, vitamin B_{12}, folate and thiamine, if available.

2 Is there a treatable brain lesion (subdural haematoma, meningioma, abscess, hydrocephalus)? Perform CT scan; if there are features to suggest chronic meningitis (e.g. TB), examine the CSF; general paralysis of the insane (GPI) is rare but if it is a clinical possibility request the plasma VDRL or TPHA (CSF VDRL, TPHA, FTA and cells and protein only if serum positive).

3 Is there a depressive pseudo-dementia? Request cognitive assessment by clinical psychologist.

Depression

Diagnosis

Exclude hypothyroidism in recent depression: carry out T4. Dexamethasone suppression test; this is used in small proportion of patients when it is unclear if there is a psychotic rather than a neurotic depression. In normal subjects a low dose of dexamethasone will suppress ACTH production, reducing the plasma cortisol for 24–48 h. In approximately 50% of patients with a depressive illness this reduction in plasma cortisol does not occur (positive). It is more likely to be positive in a psychotic rather than a neurotic depression and in more severe depression when the suicide risk is greater. Its value as a predictor of response to treatment is unclear.

Management

Electroconvulsive therapy (ECT)

Exclude patients with cardiac failure, arrhythmias, recent myocardial infarction, hypotension or other conditions contra-indicating short anaesthetic. Carry out ECG, FBC, ESR, blood biochemistry, chest X-ray and sickle cell test in Negroid patients.

Lithium carbonate therapy

Prior to therapy carry out:

1 FBC, as leucocytosis or modest leucopenia may subsequently occur.

2   ECG as T-wave depression may be induced.

3   assays on urea, creatinine and electrolytes as renal function may be impaired by lithium; check annually.

4   T4, as levels may be altered in up to 20% of patients; check annually.

5   pregnancy test, if there is a possibility of pregnancy, as lithium is contra-indicated in pregnancy (it may harm the developing foetus).

The therapeutic range is $0.5-1.2$ nmol l^{-1}. Some patients develop toxic symptoms at the top end of this range, but usually toxicity occurs above 1.5 nmol l^{-1}. At the start of treatment estimate the serum level within the first week, then at increasing intervals such as 2, 4, 6 and 8 weeks, and then every 3 months when stabilized.

Urea and T4 should be checked annually when on regular therapy.

Transient ischaemic attacks (TIA)

1   Is it TIA? Carry out EEG if possible seizure; glucose assay if possible hypoglycaemia.

2   What is the mechanism?

?cardiac arrhythmia. Carry out ECG, 24-hour ECG tape.

?carotid arterial disease. Perform Doppler duplex scanning if available; arteriography only if surgery would be considered.

?other vascular disease. Carry out ESR for vasculitis; haemoglobin, packed cell volume (PCV) for polycythaemia; white blood cell count (WBC) for leukaemia.

Subarachnoid haemorrhage

1   CT scan if available.

2   Perform LP.

3   Arteriography in confirmed subarachnoid haemorrhage as soon as it can be arranged electively in patients that may be considered for surgery and are in good neurological condition.

Chapter 7
Renal Tract Disorders

Introduction

The first section of this chapter will summarize the general symptoms which occur in renal disorders. The second section will consider individual investigations with respect to their major indications, a brief description of the procedure and any precautions, disadvantages or hazards likely to be encountered. The third part deals with common presenting features of kidney disease indicating which investigations are relevant to the management decision 'tree'.

General symptoms

The clinical manifestations of renal tract disorders are myriad. In practice, however, renal disease may be suspected in the presence of relatively few symptoms, signs and basic investigations. Common symptoms are listed in Table 7.1.

Renal pain is felt in the lumbar region but many forms of renal disease, including nephritis and tumours, may be painless or associated with a dull ache. In contrast, obstruction of the renal tract, most commonly with calculi but occasionally with blood clot or tumour fragments, leads to severe colicky pain originating in the lumbar region and radiating to the groin and sometimes into the genitalia and thigh. Infections of the lower urinary tract, cystitis and urethritis, cause frequency of micturition with dysuria. Hesitancy and a poor urinary stream are features of bladder outflow obstruction, most commonly due to prostatic disease and occasionally due to urethral strictures. The constellation of symptoms which herald renal failure includes anorexia, nausea, pruritus and lethargy.

Physical signs specific for renal tract disease are few: renal enlargement or masses, bladder enlargement, tenderness of kidneys or bladder and prostatic enlargement. Hypertension and oedema are common, although not specific for renal disease. Laboratory pointers to renal tract disease include haematuria,

Table 7.1 Common symptoms in renal tract disorders

Renal pain
Ureteric colic
Bladder pain
Pain on micturition
Frequency of micturition
A poor urinary stream
Haematuria
Oedema
Symptoms of renal failure

proteinuria, bacteriuria, elevation of serum creatinine concentration, acidosis and abnormal serum potassium.

Specific investigations

Urine

Microscopy

Cells, casts, bacteria and crystals should be sought in fresh urine, both uncentrifuged and centrifuged.

White blood cell counts (WBC) of >10 cells/high-power field of uncentrifuged urine are abnormal (one high-power field contains $0.3\,\mu l$ urine under the coverslip). Usually associated with urinary tract infection (UTI) including tuberculosis; pyuria may also be caused by chronic interstitial nephritis, stones and tumours.

Red blood cells (rbc) usually indicate a pathological process but may be physiological after strenuous exercise. Crenated dysmorphic rbcs together with casts and/or proteinuria indicate glomerular disease (glomerulonephritis); otherwise presence may be caused by many other diseases.

Casts may be rbc, hyaline or granular (Fig. 7.1). Red cell casts are found in acute or chronic glomerular disease, hyaline casts consist of Tamm Horsfall protein and are of no pathological significance, while granular casts formed of tubular cells may indicate acute tubular necrosis or acute nephritis.

Crystals, of oxalate, calcium phosphate and urate, are found in stone-formers and in normal individuals; chemical urine analysis is more reliable in diagnosing metabolic stones.

Urinalysis

The presence of protein and blood, relevant for renal disease, is detected routinely by dipstick testing.

Protein stick test is only semi-quantitative, but is highly sensitive; a negative protein stick test excludes proteinuria, except light-chain (Bence–Jones) proteinuria. Positive tests should be confirmed by quantitative urinary protein estimation.

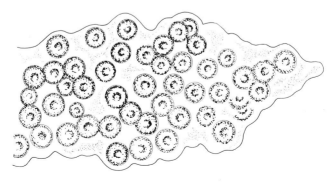

Fig. 7.1 Red cell cast.

Blood stick test is positive for intact red cells, free haemoglobin and myoglobin. Urine may appear red with negative blood stick test after eating food dyes, phenolphthalein or beetroot.

Culture

Urine may be obtained by mid-stream specimen (MSU), supra-pubic aspiration (useful in infants), bladder catheterization (undesirable unless patient needs catheter for other reasons, e.g. incontinence, retention, coma) or at cystoscopy. A positive culture of supra-pubic aspirate or fresh bladder catheter specimen always indicates UTI; interpretation of MSU depends on clinical setting, presence of wbc and purity of growth. In women with acute pyelonephritis due to Gram-negative infections a criterion of $>10^5$ organisms ml^{-1} urine provides the best differentiation between infection and contamination.

In acutely dysuric women a pure growth of as few as 10^2 organisms ml^{-1} plus wbc is likely to indicate UTI and the 10^5 organisms ml^{-1} criterion is too insensitive to be clinically useful.

In asymptomatic women $>10^5$ organisms ml^{-1} indicates UTI, but the value of treatment, except during pregnancy, is not clear.

In males, UTI is nearly always associated with $>10^5$ organisms ml^{-1} and contamination of MSU samples is less likely than in women.

Chemical analysis

Protein excretion must be quantified on a 24-hour urine collection if a dipstick shows more than a trace of protein. A loss of >200 mg per day is pathological and merits further investigation. Microalbuminuria (radio-immunoassay is needed to detect selective albumin excretion >25 mg per day) which may herald overt nephropathy in diabetics.

Protein : creatinine ratios on a single random urine sample may supplant the need for 24-hour urine collections; the ratio is related directly to quantitative proteinuria (Fig. 7.2).

Sodium excretion in health varies from almost zero to 300 mmol or more per day according to intake, and is regulated by aldosterone and atrial natriuretic peptide. Inappropriate sodium excretion ('salt-losing nephropathy') typifies tubulo-interstitial diseases such as obstructive uropathy, chronic pyelonephritis and analgesic nephropathy. In oliguric states urinary sodium concentration of <20 mmol l^{-1} signifies renal hypoperfusion, while a greater loss suggests acute tubular necrosis or some other form of intrinsic renal failure.

Potassium concentration in the urine cannot be reduced below 20 mmol l^{-1}, even in the face of hypokalaemia; urinary K^+ >30 mmol l^{-1} with a plasma K^+ <3.4 mmol l^{-1} suggests renal potassium wasting, as a result of adrenocorticoid excess (Cushing's or Conn's syndrome), primary renal disorders (including renal tubular acidosis and Bartter's syndrome), or diuretic use (and abuse).

Urinary pH varies widely according to diet and metabolism. An acid urine in the face of systemic acidosis is physiological; urine pH >5.3, when plasma bicarbonate or pH is low, indicates a metabolic acidosis of renal origin, as a result of a reduced glomerular filtration rate (GFR) (uraemic acidosis) or of renal

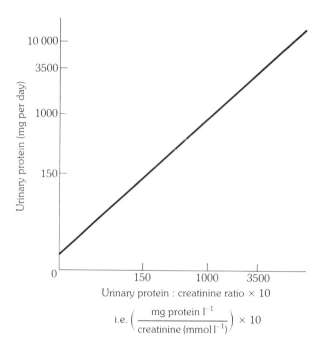

Fig. 7.2 Relationship between urinary protein : creatinine ratio and 24-hour urinary protein output. After Shaw, A.B. *et al.* (1983) *British Medical Journal*, **287**, 929–32.

tubular acidosis. An acid load test may be necessary but not if urine pH is <5.3, while plasma HCO_3 concentration is <20 mmol l^{-1}.

Acid load test is performed by giving ammonium chloride 100 mg kg^{-1} and measuring urinary pH and plasma bicarbonate for 8 h. Failure to acidify the urine below pH 5.3 in the face of a plasma bicarbonate concentration of <20 mmol l^{-1} indicates renal tubular acidosis.

Urinary osmolality depends on fluid intake and is regulated by antidiuretic hormone. Diabetes insipidus is diagnosed when urinary osmolality fails to rise above 750 mosmol kg^{-1} during a period of water deprivation sufficient to allow body weight to fall by 2 kg. Pituitary diabetes insipidus can be corrected by administration of desmopressin 4 µg i.m.; the nephrogenic form, resulting from tubular dysfunction, will fail to show urinary concentration after desmopressin. A water deprivation test is unnecessary if a random (or preferably, overnight) urine sample has an osmolality >550 mosmol kg^{-1}. Osmolality is osmotic pressure measured in osmoles (osmol) or milliosmoles (mosmol) per kilogram of water, whereas osmolarity expresses the pressure in osmoles per litre of solution. Osmolality is generally used for body fluids; normal serum osmolality is around 290 mosmol.

In oliguric patients urine osmolality is useful; when increased, poor renal perfusion (pre-renal failure) is likely, but if normal, intrinsic renal failure (e.g. acute tubular necrosis) may have developed. Only in the former case is the ratio of the osmolalities noted in urine and plasma (u : p ratio >1.5).

Calcium excretion (normal <7.5 mmol per day) is increased in hypercalcaemic states (hyperparathyroidism, disseminated malignancy, sarcoidosis, vitamin D excess, milk-alkali syndrome). Idiopathic hypercalciuria is present when plasma calcium is normal but urinary calcium is increased; this is associated with some recurrent stone-formers.

Oxalate and urate are less often measured in stone-formers, but may relate more closely to the tendency to urinary supersaturation and stone formation.

Urea concentration in urine may be measured in patients with oliguria. In patients with pre-renal failure the ratio of urinary urea concentration : serum urea concentration is at least 10 : 1, whereas in intrinsic renal failure the ratio is considerably reduced.

Amino acids are not normally present in excessive quantities in the urine. Fanconi syndrome is characterized by increased urinary amino acid excretion (detected by chromatography) and proximal tubular bicarbonate wasting. Cystinuria results in recurrent stone formation and loss of cystine, ornithine, lysine and arginine in the urine.

Light-chain immunoglobulin fractions (previously known as Bence–Jones protein) appear in the urine in patients with myeloma and are detected by immuno-electrophoresis.

Clearance measurements can be made for any substance using the formula UV/P, where U is the urinary concentration of the substance studied, P is its plasma concentration and V the urine volume in a specified time. Inulin clearance is the reference standard for GFR as inulin is freely filtered, and undergoes neither secretion nor re-absorption by tubules. Measurement is cumbersome and unsuited to clinical practice; [^{51}Cr]EDTA clearance provides a more accurate but expensive method (see p.140). Creatinine clearance is the time-honoured measure of GFR, but is invalid at low GFR because of tubular secretion of creatinine. Furthermore, timed urine collections are often inaccurate. In the steady state, $U_{Cr}V$ equals endogenous production, and is purely dependent on muscle bulk. Thus, for an individual, creatinine clearance is inversely related to plasma creatinine concentration and serial measurements of creatinine clearance provide little extra information over plasma creatinine. Formulae can be used to calculate creatinine clearance based on plasma creatinine, age and weight.

Males

$$\text{GFR (ml s}^{-1}) = \frac{(140 - \text{age}) \times \text{weight (kg)}}{49 \times \text{creatinine } (\mu \text{mol l}^{-1})}.$$

Females
Calculate as for males and multiply by 0.85.

Children

$$\text{GFR (ml.min}^{-1}.1.73 \text{ m}^{-2}) = \frac{40 \times \text{height (cm)}}{\text{creatinine (}\mu\text{mol l}^{-1})}.$$

Increases in serum creatinine concentration above laboratory references ranges may, however, require at least a 50% reduction in GFR. If a slight reduction in GFR is suspected in a patient with serum creatinine concentrations within the normal range this may be assessed by [^{51}Cr]EDTA or creatinine clearance techniques.

Blood tests

Biochemistry

Serum urea concentration is a poor guide to renal function because it is influenced by many factors, including GFR, protein intake, catabolism, gastro-intestinal haemorrhage, diuretic therapy and heart failure. A normal serum urea concentration is, in general, an indication of normal kidney function if the patient is clinically well on a normal diet; otherwise it is difficult to interpret.

Serum creatinine concentration is the simplest and most readily available guide to kidney function. For any given individual, plasma creatinine is inversely related to creatinine clearance provided that muscle bulk (and hence endogenous creatinine generation) is stable. Progression of kidney disease is best assessed by serial creatinine measurements.

A doubling of plasma creatinine indicates a halving of kidney function; however, more than 50% of renal function is lost before serum creatinine concentration increases above normal.

When serum concentrations of both urea and creatinine are measured, additional diagnostic information may be available. Both concentrations may increase equally or the concentration of one substance may increase out of proportion to the other. For example, when a patient has a serum urea concentration of 45 mmol l^{-1} and a serum creatinine concentration of $200 \text{ }\mu\text{mol l}^{-1}$, serum urea is elevated to a greater extent than creatinine; the serum urea concentration of 45 mmol l^{-1} is more than six times the upper limit of normal (7 mmol l^{-1}), while the serum creatinine concentration $(200 \text{ }\mu\text{mol l}^{-1})$ is only twice the normal value of $100 \text{ }\mu\text{mol l}^{-1}$.

1 Serum urea and creatinine concentrations are equally elevated in established renal failure, both acute and chronic.

2 Serum creatinine may be raised out of proportion to urea because of:

(a) rhabdomyolysis, which is associated with elevated serum levels of muscle enzymes, or

(b) long-term dialysis treatment because urea molecules are smaller and more readily removed by dialysis than are creatinine molecules.

Very occasionally, drugs such as aspirin or cotrimoxazole cause a similar, but lesser, effect by blocking the tubular secretion of creatinine.

3 Serum urea may also be raised out of proportion to creatinine because of:

(a) Salt and water depletion of diuretic therapy.

(b) Dietary protein load or gastro-intestinal haemorrhage.

(c) Hypercatabolic states resulting from trauma and infection of drugs such as corticosteroids or tetracyclines (which have an anti-anabolic effect).

4 Serum urea concentration may be decreased out of proportion to creatinine in liver failure, low protein diet, high fluid intake and pregnancy.

Serum sodium concentration is generally normal in kidney disease, but may vary in diseases mediated by kidney function, e.g. hypernatraemia in diabetes insipidus, hyponatraemia in inappropriate antidiuretic hormone (ADH) secretion.

Serum potassium concentration rarely increases above normal values in kidney failure until GFR falls below 20 ml min^{-1}. Occasionally hyperkalaemia is found with acidosis (type IV renal tubular acidosis) at more modest degrees of renal impairment. Hypokalaemia is characteristic of proximal and distal renal tubular acidosis and Bartter's syndrome. Hypokalaemia and acid urine indicate non-renal potassium loss or deficiency.

Serum bicarbonate concentration provides a simple guide to acid base status. The formula

$$(25 - \text{plasma bicarbonate}) \times \frac{\text{body weight (kg)}}{3}$$

is a valuable guide to total body bicarbonate deficit (in mmol). Correction of acidosis will reverse associated hyperkalaemia. Acidosis in renal disease is either due to renal impairment or tubular disorders; urine pH is >5.4 in renal acidosis, but <5.4 with acidosis from other causes (e.g. ketoacidosis, lactic acidosis).

Albumin is low in nephrotic syndrome, usually inversely proportional to the severity of the glomerular protein leak.

Globulin levels are high in many conditions; electrophoresis indicates paraproteins and quantifies individual immunoglobulin classes.

Serum calcium and phosphate concentrations become abnormal in renal impairment as a result of deficient phosphate excretion and impaired renal 1-alpha hydroxylation of vitamin D. Total calcium is low in hypoalbuminaemia. Ionized calcium (calculated or directly measured) provides a better assessment of calcium status.

Serum alkaline phosphatase activity is characteristically elevated in renal osteodystrophy, but is an insensitive marker. Parathyroid hormone (PTH) assays are preferable.

Serum urate concentrations parallel creatinine as renal failure progresses. Disproportionate elevation of urate indicates primary or secondary hyperuricaemia.

Haematology

Haemoglobin falls as renal failure progresses, otherwise it is seldom of diagnostic value in renal disease. Immune haemolytic anaemia is characteristic of systemic lupus erythematosus (SLE). Microangiopathic haemolytic anaemia may occur in haemolytic uraemic syndrome, thrombotic thrombocytopenic purpura, accelerated hypertension and some cases of vascular transplant rejection.

White cell count is elevated, usually polymorphonuclear leucocytes, in polyarteritis and Wegener's granulomatosis; occasionally an eosinophilia is present. Leucopenia is commonly found in SLE.

Platelets fall in disseminated intravascular coagulation (DIC), which is common in acute renal failure because of sepsis. Immune thrombocytopenia is found in SLE.

Sedimentation rate is typically elevated in collagen vascular diseases and reflects disease activity. It may also be elevated in chronic renal failure and nephrotic syndrome (because of increased plasma fibrinogen concentration).

Immunological tests

Antinuclear antibodies characterize SLE, but false positives occur; antibodies to native double-stranded DNA are more specific, but less sensitive.

Complement is activated in several renal diseases. C3 is low in the acute phase of post-streptococcal glomerulonephritis, and rises with recovery. In contrast, C3 is persistently low in mesangiocapillary glomerulonephritis. Depression of both C3 and C4 occurs in SLE, but also in chronic infections which may present with renal disease, e.g. infective endocarditis.

Immunoglobulin (Ig) estimation and immunoelectrophoresis may show polyclonal Ig elevation in collagen vascular diseases, or reveal a monoclonal band in myeloma. Immune paresis without a band is common in primary amyloidosis.

Antistreptolysin-O titre (ASOT) should be measured in acute nephritic illnesses.

Immune complexes (assayed by a variety of methods) can be found in many glomerular diseases, but at present these are of research interest only.

Cryoglobulins are immune complexes that precipitate on cooling blood or serum and are found in SLE, lymphomas, leukaemias and essential cryoglobulinaemia.

Coagulation studies must be normal before renal biopsy. Prolonged prothrombin time and/or activated partial thromboplastin time characterizes DIC.

Microbiological tests

Blood cultures are essential for the diagnosis of endocarditis which may present as nephritis.

Serology can provide evidence of previous infection by many agents which may be implicated in the aetiology of various glomerular diseases (e.g. *Treponema pallidum* haemagglutination assay, TPHA).

Diagnostic imaging

X-rays

Plain films may show stones and renal size.

Intravenous urogram (IVU) or pyelogram (IVP) remains the best initial study in evaluation of renal disease. It identifies and characterizes renal parenchymal disease and provides an indication of renal function. Cysts, tumours, scars, papillary necrosis, obstruction, pelvi-ureteric filling defects, stones and structural anomalies may all be demonstrated. Bladder films pre- and post-micturition may show diverticulae, ureteroceles, stones, neoplasms, prostatic obstruction and residual urine. Proper bowel preparation is essential; dehydration must be avoided in patients with renal impairment, diabetes and suspected myeloma. High doses of contrast are needed in renal impairment and are usually administered by intravenous infusion; good quality films are unlikely if plasma creatinine $>500 \, \mu mol \, l^{-1}$. An increasingly dense nephrogram is characteristic of acute tubular necrosis; late films for the diagnosis of obstruction are virtually obsolete with the use of ultrasound (q.v.). Tomography may help in the evaluation of renal outlines and masses, particularly when bowel shadows obscure detail. Minor reactions to contrast agents are common; bronchospasm or urticaria affects 1.5%, while severe life-threatening reactions affect one in 2500 patients.

Retrograde pyelograph is an invasive, combined urological/radiological investigation used principally to demonstrate the causes of ureteric obstructions shown in IVU or ultrasound. Occasionally it is of value in excluding obstruction or in visualizing filling defects not clearly seen on IVU. It is also useful in unilateral ureteric bleeding and in excluding obstruction in unilateral non-functioning kidneys but has largely been replaced by antegrade pyelography.

Antegrade pyelography involves puncturing the renal pelvis or a calix and injecting contrast to allow visualization of the collecting system. The pelvi-caliceal system must first be shown on ultrasound to be dilated, and puncture is guided by ultrasound localization. The technique is often combined with percutaneous nephrostomy to allow drainage of an obstructed kidney and permit pressure-flow studies in the evaluation of hydro-ureter and hydronephrosis. It is indicated when retrograde pyelography is impossible or unsafe.

Micturating cystography (MCU) and urethrography are invasive techniques used to evaluate vesico-ureteric reflux, bladder emptying and urethral lesions such as valves and stenoses.

Arteriography is conventionally performed via a femoral arterial puncture, but digital subtraction techniques allow arterial visualization after intravenous contrast injection in most patients. Aortography is usually sufficient to show renal artery stenosis; selective arteriography may be necessary to visualize tumours, arteriovenous malformations, and is essential for such interventional techniques as angioplasty and embolization. Ultrasound and CT scanning have largely replaced arteriography in the diagnosis of most renal masses. Venography may occasionally assist in the evaluation of some renal tumours and the diagnosis of renal vein thrombosis (rare).

Computerized tomography has particular value in the diagnosis of renal masses, perinephric lesions and poorly or non-functioning kidneys. It is preceded by IVU and ultrasound.

Other X-rays may be helpful in the evaluation of renal disease, e.g. chest X-ray in systemic disorders, such as collagen vascular disease, or bone X-rays in renal osteodystrophy.

Ultrasound

Renal ultrasound has revolutionized the management of two main problems: the patient with renal failure; and the evaluation of renal masses. Renal ultrasound clearly demonstrates pelvi-caliceal dilatation and renal size, even in the absence of kidney function, and thereby divides patients with renal failure into three groups: those with (i) obstructions; (ii)small kidneys (chronic renal failure); and (iii) acute parenchymal disease. Rarely, the ultrasound appearances of polycystic disease may be mistaken for hydronephrosis. Masses can be shown to be solid (tumours) or cystic (benign). In 50% of patients sufficient corticomedullary definition permits a tentative diagnosis of a variety of conditions, including suppurative pyelonephritis, infarction and diffuse cortical disease.

Radioisotopic imaging

The main place of renal isotope scanning is to provide functional measurements to complement the structural information provided by X-rays and ultrasound. In addition, structural information can be provided in those allergic to X-ray contrast or with renal failure. The small dose of radiotracer permits repeated evaluation of patients to assess the course of renal disease.

Technetium-99m diethylenetriamine penta-acetic acid (^{99m}Tc-DTPA) is the radiopharmaceutical used for standard isotope renography. It provides a guide to relative renal blood flow, relative renal function and the presence of obstruction. The agent is usually cleared from the kidney by 30 min and progressive accumulation beyond this time suggests obstruction.

Technetium-99m dimercaptosuccinate (^{99m}Tc-DMSA) is an agent with negligible urinary excretion; hence, it is of no value in imaging the collecting system or assessing obstruction. Its main value is the ability to produce high-quality cortical images to demonstrate infarcts, scars, cysts, tumours, etc. Divided renal function (i.e. the function of each kidney) can be measured non-invasively because the images relate to functional renal mass.

Iodine-131 ortho-iodohippuric acid (^{131}I-hippuran) has a renal plasma clearance of over 85%, and is therefore useful in estimating effective renal plasma flow. The high alpha and beta emissions of ^{131}I detract from its clinical value, and ^{123}I is a preferable label for hippuran, although less readily available.

Chromium-51 ethylene diamine tetra-acetic acid (^{51}Cr-EDTA) is used to determine GFR. A single injection followed by one or several timed blood samples will enable GFR to be calculated as accurately, and more conveniently, than inulin clearance. The method is inaccurate in gross oedema (e.g. untreated nephrotic syndrome).

Histopathology

In addition to renal biopsy, histological examination of other organs (skin, muscle, gum, rectum) aids in the evaluation of systemic diseases, involving the kidney, such as amyloidosis, vasculitis, anaphylactoid purpura, etc.

Renal biopsy

Indications

Nephrotic syndrome, unresolved or atypical acute nephritis, persistent haematuria and/or proteinuria, multisystem disease involving the kidney, acute or chronic renal impairment after exclusion of obstruction or bilaterally small kidneys (by ultrasound scanning (USS) or radiology).

Preparations

IVU or renogram to demonstrate function of both kidneys (percutaneous biopsy of a single functioning kidney is contra-indicated as open biopsy is less hazardous). Normal prothrombin time and partial thromboplastin time; normal platelet count, normal template bleeding time if patient uraemic. Group and save serum (cross-matching of blood not necessary). Adequate premedication to provide sedation and analgesia, but allow patient co-operation.

Procedure

Biopsy performed after ultrasound localization of lower pole of right or left kidney, or under X-ray screening of the kidneys with or without contrast. Specimens sent for light microscopy (formalin-fixed), immunofluorescent examination (fresh or frozen) and electron microscopy (fresh or xylol-fixed).

Aftercare

Pulse and blood pressure monitored every 15 min for 1 h, every 30 min for 2 h, hourly for 4 h and then 4-hourly. Hypotension during/after biopsy may be due to vasovagal syncope (bradycardia) or haemorrhage (tachycardia).

Haemorrhage may be perirenal or into the urinary tract. Water diuresis after biopsy minimizes the risk of clot obstruction in the event of urinary tract bleeding. Risk of bleeding requiring transfusion <5%; risk of continued bleeding requiring nephrectomy or renal embolization <1:1000. Risk of death negligible.

Interpretation

Light microscopy will distinguish between tubulo-interstitial diseases, vascular disorders and glomerular pathology. Immunofluorescent microscopy reveals the presence and pattern of immunoglobulin and fibrin deposition, while electron microscopy defines precisely the location of immune deposits.

Cytology

Cytological examination of the urine may be useful in the diagnosis of urothelial malignancy. Fluid obtained from renal cyst puncture can be examined for malignant cells. Urinary red cell morphology may distinguish between glomerular bleeding (crenated, fragmented cells) and urothelial or other renal tract bleeding (normal red cells).

Diagnostic approach

This section lists a suggested order of investigations for a variety of presentations of urinary tract disease. Basic tests should be requested before proceeding to the next level of investigation, or to an alternative decision 'tree'. The previous section can be referred to for specific details of tests and interpretation. The righthand column indicates diagnosis to be considered (or occasionally excluded) by the investigations listed.

Symptoms

Renal pain
1 MSU · · · · · · · · · · · · · · · · · · · UTI
  Urine microscopy ? rbc · · · · · Stones, tumour, glomerulonephritis (occasionally), loin pain/haematuria syndrome, renal arteriovenous malformation
2 IVU · · · · · · · · · · · · · · · · · · · Stones, tumour
3 Follow protocols for stones, UTI, space-occupying lesion, etc.
4 Consider biliary, colonic, spinal or gynaecologic cause for symptoms if 1 and 2 are negative.

Bladder pain/urethral pain
1 MSU · · · · · · · · · · · · · · · · · · · UTI (Note importance of low colony counts when symptoms present)
  Urine microscopy ? rbc · · · · · Bladder cancer
             ? wbc · · · · · TB bladder (send early morning urine specimen)
  Urethral smear · · · · · · · · · · · Gonorrhoea, chlamydial urethritis
2 Cysto-urethroscopy with/without biopsy · · · · · · · Bladder cancer, TB bladder, bladder stone, interstitial cystitis
NB See p. 145 for investigation of bacteriuria.

Frequency of micturition
1 Voided volume · · · · · · · · · · · If large, see polyuria protocol; if small, continue
2 MSU · · · · · · · · · · · · · · · · · · · UTI
  Rectal examination · · · · · · · · Prostatic enlargement (q.v.)
3 Ultrasound bladder post-micturition · · · · · · · · · · Bladder outlet obstruction
4 Urine flow measurement · · · · Bladder outlet obstruction
5 Full urodynamic investigation including cystoscopy · · · · · · · Neuropathic bladder disorders, bladder tumours, stones, etc.

True polyuria (large voided volumes)
1 24-hour urine volume
2 Urine/blood glucose · · · · · · · Diabetes mellitus
3 Serum, creatinine, potassium, sodium, calcium · · · · · · · · · · Renal failure, electrolyte disorders, diabetes insipidus
4 Overnight urine osmolality · · · Primary polydipsia
5 IVP, renogram or ultrasound · partial obstruction
6 Water deprivation test · · · · · · Diabetes insipidus
7 Response to pitressin · · · · · · Nephrogenic or pituitary cause

Poor urine flow
1 Rectal examination · · · · · · · · Prostatic disease

	Urine flow measurement	To confirm problem
2	Ultrasound bladder after micturition	Bladder outlet obstruction, prostate can be seen on scan
3	Cysto-urethroscopy	Urethral strictures, valves, stones
4	Urethrography	As above
5	Urodynamic studies	Neuropathic bladder disorders

Frank (macroscopic) haematuria

1	Stick test for blood	Beetrooturia
	Urine microscopy	True haematuria
	Exclude sickle cell disease	Haemoglobinuria
2	IVU	Tumours, stones
	Serum creatinine	Renal damage
3	Cystoscopy	Bladder cancer or stone
4	Follow protocol for microscopic haematuria if no diagnosis	
5	Consider renal angiography	Arteriovenous malformation, renal embolism

Ureteric colic/renal colic/renal stones

1	Plain abdominal film	To confirm diagnosis
2	IVU (emergency if diagnostic doubt)	As above
3	MSU : microscopy	Phosphate stones ('staghorn calculi') associated with *Proteus* infections
4	Chemical stone analysis	Metabolic stone disorders
5	Serum calcium, phosphate, urate	As above
6	24-hour urine analysis for calcium phosphate, oxalate	As above
7	Dietary history	
8	Serum parathyroid hormone; exclude enteric hyperoxaluria; exclude causes of urate overproduction	If above tests point to specific metabolic disorders

Oedema

Oedema is *not* a cardinal feature of kidney disease; protocols for proteinuria, hypertension or renal impairment should be followed.

Signs

Renal enlargement/masses

1	IVU	Hydronephrosis, cysts, space-occupying
	Ultrasound	lesions
	(both not essential, diagnosis, may be made by either test,	

but investigations are complementary)

Serum creatinine — Polycystic disease, obstructive uropathy

2 Follow protocol for space-occupying lesions or hydronephrosis

Renal space-occupying lesion

1 Ultrasound — Cystic or solid lesions
2 CT—if solid lesion consider angiography — Tumours
3 Cyst puncture and contrast studies if irregular wall to cyst — Necrotic tumours

Hydronephrosis

1 Ultrasound ureters/bladder — Defines level of obstruction
2 Antegrade pyelography of obstructions at ureteric levels and caliceal dilation permits percutaneous puncture
3 Retrograde pyelography
4 CT scanning — Pelvic malignant disease

Bladder enlargement

1 Ultrasound (to confirm diagnosis)
2 Urine flow — Bladder outlet obstruction
3 Cystoscopy — Tumours, stones

Prostatic enlargement

1 Serum creatinine — Obstructive uropathy
2 Acid phosphatase — Carcinoma
(Now being superseded by prostate-specific antigen)
3 Ultrasound kidneys and bladder — Obstruction

Hypertension

Although renal disease is the commonest cause of secondary hypertension, a treatable lesion (e.g. renal artery stenosis) is rarely found. In general, it is better to investigate for associated risk factors for vascular disease (e.g. hyperlipidaemia, left ventricular hypertrophy) rather than to search for a cause for hypertension.

1 Urinalysis — Renal cause or secondary renal damage
Serum creatinine — As above
Serum electrolytes — Conn's syndrome, Cushing's syndrome
ECG, chest X-ray — Evidence of left ventricular hypertrophy

2 IVU if <35 years of age and no family history *or* pointer to renal disease from 1 *or* hypertension resistant to two drug treatment.

3 Renal angiography (preferably digital subtraction angiography) if renal bruit *or* declining renal function with good BP control and no evidence of a renal cause on 1 and 2 *or* BP resistant to three drug treatment.

Renography (isotope) is not useful in excluding renal artery stenosis: false negative results are too frequent.

Laboratory abnormalities

Bacteriuria

1 Repeat MSU a week after treatment.

2 IVU — Structural abnormalities of
- males — renal tract, e.g. stones,
- children — obstruction, reflux
- recurrent attacks in women
- renal impairment
- severe clinical pyelonephritis

3 Renal ultrasound if recurrent pyelonephritis — Renal suppuration

4 Micturating cysto-urethrography — If IVU or history suggests reflux

Proteinuria (stick positive)

1 Recurrent overnight urine sample — Orthostatic proteinuria

2 MSU — UTI

3 Quantitative urine protein (24-hour sample or protein/creatinine ratio), urine microscopy (? rbc), serum creatinine, albumin, blood pressure, microscopy for casts

4 FBC, ESR
IVU — Structural lesions
Blood glucose — Diabetes mellitus

5 ASOT
Autoantibodies — SLE
Immunoglobulins — Myeloma
Urinary free light-chains
Complement levels
Neutrophil anticytoplasmic antibodies — Polyarteritis nodosa, Wegener's granulomatosis

6 Renal biopsy if proteinuria 3 g/day *or* renal impairment *or* hypertension *or* proteinuria 1–3 g/day with rbcs

Microscopic haematuria

If patient >40 years of age, proceed as for macroscopic haematuria, unless microscopy shows casts.

If casts present, or patient <40 years of age:

1 IVU
   Serum creatinine
2 Follow proteinuria protocol   Glomerular disease
3 Chest X-ray, ears, nose and   Systemic vasculitis
   throat examination, glomerular
   basement membrane antibodies,
   neutrophil anticytoplasmic
   antibodies

Elevated serum creatinine

1 Is level appropriate for patient's
   muscle bulk ?
2 Measure urine output (catheter
   if necessary)
3 Repeat immediately and in   ? rising or static
   1 week
4 Consider clinical state of
   patient; *either* precipitating
   illness such as sepsis, shock,
   hypovolaemia, major surgery,
   major trauma *or* no identifiable
   reason for renal failure *if*
   precipitating illness present
5 Urine/plasma osmolality   Low in acute tubular necrosis (ATN)
   Urine sodium concentration   Elevated in ATN; low in pre-renal
                                        azotaemia

   Measure central venous   Hypovolaemia
   pressure/primary capillary
   wedge pressure/BP
   Send blood cultures (assume
   sepsis present) *if* 'unexpected'
   uraemia
6 IVU if creatinine <400–500 μmol l^{-1}
   USS if creatinine >500 μmol l^{-1}
   $\pm$ DTPA renogram
   $\pm$ DMSA renogram
7 Follow investigations for
   hydronephrosis, if present
8 Renal angiography if no
   perfusion on renography
9 Renal biopsy for normal-sized   Intrinsic renal diseases,
   non-obstructed kidneys   e.g. glomerulonephritis, interstitial
                                          nephritis

Systemic acidosis

1 Arterial blood gases — Metabolic or respiratory
2 Urine sugar, ketones, blood sugar — Ketoacidosis
3 Serum creatinine — Renal failure
4 Salicylate level — Poisoning
5 Plasma lactate — Lactic acidosis
6 Urine pH — Normally <5.3 if plasma HCO_3, <20 mmol l^{-1}
7 Acid load test (q.v.)

Hypokalaemia

1 Drug history — Diuretics
  Check blood pressure — Conn's syndrome
2 Urine pH — Acid urine suggests non-renal potassium loss
3 Urine potassium concentration — >30 mmol l^{-1} suggests renal, potassium wasting; 20–30 mmol l^{-1} is minimal urine potassium concentration
4 If renal potassium losing state — Reconsider diuretic use/abuse
  Exclude renal tubular acidosis
  Measure plasma renin/aldosterone

Hyperkalaemia

1 Serum bicarbonate — Acidosis—cellular potassium leak
2 Serum sodium — Addison's disease
  Blood pressure
3 Blood glucose — Diabetes mellitus
4 Serum creatinine — Renal failure

Chapter 8
Rheumatology

Introduction

The investigation of any rheumatic disease must begin with a comprehensive clinical history and general medical examination. In many patients an accurate diagnosis and assessment of disease activity can be made at that point, so that practical procedures and laboratory data may not be necessary. A thorough practical knowledge of history taking and ability to examine the locomotor system is essential.

Patients do present with symptoms and signs where a precise diagnosis is not clear but it may be suspected that the problems will be self-limiting or might develop into a more typical form. Time is a crucial factor in establishing the diagnosis, tempo and direction of such situations. The important clinical decision at presentation, therefore, is whether immediate investigation is indicated. It is often appropriate to allow an observation interval of 6 weeks before embarking on laboratory tests and, during this time, self-resolving conditions will settle or suspected diagnoses become more apparent. There are several exceptions which demand immediate attention:

1 Severe symptoms in a single joint. This may occur in gout or sepsis and requires investigation, principally aspiration.

2 A systemically ill patient with significant muscular weakness or where several organ systems are involved. A systemic connective tissue disease, tuberculosis or malignancy may present in this way.

3 Associated neurological symptoms, e.g. carpal tunnel syndrome, cervical nerve entrapment or sciatica.

4 Symptoms of headache, scalp tenderness, jaw claudication, general debility and where giant cell arteritis is a possibility (visual loss is a late and usually permanent complication).

5 Significant trauma requiring orthopaedic attention. Fracture, dislocation or ligamentous tear.

General symptoms

Symptoms in rheumatology must be interpreted in relation to their clinical setting. Thus, a complaint in a middle-aged woman of symmetrical peripheral arthralgia with early morning stiffness and evidence of synovitis on examination would prompt investigation of rheumatoid arthritis. A younger patient with arthritis of knees or ankles together with dactylitis and urethritis may be suffering from Reiter's syndrome. Conversely, an older person with stiffness in the knees or hips, particularly after resting, and pain when moving the joints, with no evidence of active inflammation, would suggest osteoarthritis and X-rays would be the appropriate investigation. A middle-aged, overweight, hypertensive man

148

with sudden acute pain in the hallux, typifies gout. The possibility of infection of the joint should always be considered in patients who present acutely with monoarthritis.

Not all rheumatological disorders necessarily present with joint pain. Giant cell arteritis is one example in which headache and scalp tenderness may be the dominant complaints. The failure to recognize this condition may cost the patient his or her eyesight. Polyarteritis nodosa is a vasculitis with systemic implications and diverse symptoms. Furthermore, the joint manifestation of systemic disorders such as systemic lupus erythematosus (SLE) may not be present at the time of consultation when the diagnosis must be suspected on the basis of other symptoms or signs including skin rashes, pleuritic pain and neurological features.

Finally, arthralgia may be a feature of a variety of disorders. For example, it occurs early in the course of type B hepatitis, with other viral infections such as Rubella.

Specific investigations

When it has been established that the patient does not have a self-resolving rheumatic problem but requires further investigation, then it is necessary to consider the range of tests available and request according to the likely value of results. The principal investigations involve blood tests (haematology, biochemistry and immunology), radiology, microbiology, synovial fluid analysis and, sometimes, synovial biopsy and radioisotope scanning.

Haematology tests

Full blood count

A full blood count (FBC) should be performed in most patients, particularly those presenting with inflammatory arthritis. A moderate degree of anaemia is common with a haemoglobin level usually in the range $8-12$ g dl^{-1}. Although classically described as being a normochromic, normocytic anaemia, most patients have hypochromic red cells (mean corpuscular haemoglobin (MCH) <27 pg).

Hypochromia and microcytosis suggest iron deficiency. Assessment of iron status in patients with rheumatoid arthritis is difficult. With active disease, serum iron levels are often low and iron binding capacity equivocal, even in the absence of iron deficiency. Serum ferritin behaves as an acute phase reactant and may be unreliably raised, although a low ferritin level ($<10\,\mu g\,l^{-1}$) does strongly suggest iron deficiency. In practice, interpretation of the blood count ($\pm$ ferritin level) is made, then the response to oral iron monitored.

The most frequent cause of iron deficiency is blood loss from the upper gastro-intestinal tract; it is important to ask about dyspepsia and also to check drug treatment. All non-steroidal anti-inflammatory drugs (NSAID) may cause blood loss, ranging from microscopic to the frank haemorrhage of a peptic ulcer. Gastroscopy is often used to look for mucosal damage.

Occasionally, a co-existent bowel tumour may cause or contribute to iron deficiency.

Haematological monitoring of treatment with gold, penicillamine or potentially marrow-toxic drugs involves a regular (initially fortnightly, then monthly after 3 months) FBC looking for thrombocytopenia (usually due to peripheral platelet destruction), agranulocytosis or, disastrously, aplasia. Neutropenia can occur during the initial months of treatment with sulphasalazine. Neutrophilia and lymphopenia may accompany systemic glucocorticoid administration.

Erythrocyte sedimentation rate (ESR) and viscosity

The ESR is routinely estimated, providing a non-specific measure of disease activity in inflammatory arthritis. Typically, the ESR is high (>50 mm hr^{-1}) in active rheumatoid arthritis and associated with a normochromic anaemia and thrombocytosis. Occasionally, a normal ESR occurs despite clinically active inflammation. Plasma viscosity has replaced the ESR in some laboratories. It is an automated process; the results are not affected by age, sex or haematocrit and the normal range is 1.5–1.72 cP.

The ESR and polymorph count are raised in infection, gout and vasculitis. In the latter, e.g. polyarteritis nodosa, the ESR and polymorph count can be the best guide to disease activity and treatment.

Biochemistry tests

Renal

The kidney may be involved as part of a systemic connective tissue disease or renal damage can occur as a result of drug treatment.

Electrolytes, including urea and creatinine, are routinely measured. Renal impairment can reduce excretion of drugs, leading to accumulation which is a particular risk for the elderly. NSAIDs can be associated with deteriorating renal function and prolonged, severe toxicity may result in papillary necrosis. Proteinuria with a heavy deposit of leucocytes suggests analgesic nephropathy.

Dipstick testing of urine is regularly performed and followed by microscopy if abnormal constituents are present. Creatinine clearance may be estimated if renal function is deteriorating and 24-hour protein excretion quantified in patients with heavy proteinuria (1+ or more) on stick testing. Occasionally, urate excretion is measured in a gouty patient.

Microscopic haematuria can present a dilemma. The abnormality may be caused by menstrual contamination, local infection, glomerular disease, drug treatment (second or third line agents) or urinary tract pathology. A 'haemolysed trace' on the dipstick is probably not significant but if there is any doubt, or red cells are seen on microscopy, then renal ultrasound intravenous urography (IVU) followed by cystoscopy must be performed.

Hepatic

Liver function tests are frequently estimated. There may be intrinsic hepatic disease or a drug related abnormality. It is essential to know baseline levels before treatment with a potentially hepatotoxic agent. Liver biopsy may be indicated if there is any doubt. The alkaline phosphatase enzyme is often raised in rheumatic disorders, sometimes as a 'non-specific' finding, and a liver or bone source may be differentiated by estimating the gamma-glutamyl transpeptidase (γGT) level. Active Paget's disease and osteomalacia result in raised alkaline phosphatase levels.

Uric acid

Serum urate is raised in the majority of gouty patients at the time of acute presentation, although the only certain diagnostic test is demonstration of negatively birefringent needle-shaped crystals in synovial fluid using a polarizing microscope. A modest elevation of serum urate level is not necessarily evidence for gout and may be due to obesity or exogenous agents, including diuretics and alcohol.

Miscellaneous

Non-specific rheumatic complaints may be due to hypothyroidism or hyperparathyroidism. Hyperparathyroidism is sometimes diagnosed fortuitously via the laboratory through an unrequested serum calcium result.

Other biochemical tests include creatine kinase, which is usually elevated in polymyositis; angiotensin converting enzyme level, which may reflect disease activity in systemic sarcoidosis; and urine amino acid chromatography for evidence of the amino acid metabolism disease—homocystinuria (rare). Ochronosis (the clinical manifestation of alcaptonuria) results from deposition of homogentisic acid in various tissues, especially cartilage. Homogentisic acid in the urine turns a dark colour on oxidation or addition of alkali.

Microbiology

Polyarthritis may occur during certain viral infections, the most common being rubella, type B hepatitis, mumps and infectious mononucleosis. Serological evidence can be used to confirm infection but the arthritis is usually mild and self-limiting.

Synovial fluid specimens may be sent for microbiological examination. This should include Gram stain and culture for the investigation of bacterial infection.

Immunology tests

Rheumatoid factor (RF)

For routine clinical purposes the RF refers to an IgM antibody directed against altered IgG molecules. Detection is by an agglutination test and the nature of substrate particles determines the name of the test (sheep red blood cells for Rose-Waaler and latex for the RA latex).

The rheumatoid factor test is not a specific test, being positive in many connective tissue diseases apart from rheumatoid arthritis, and also in other chronic disorders (Table 8.1). Positive results are found in about 70% of patients with active rheumatoid arthritis. A high titre shows correlation with disease activity, and particularly systemic complications like nodules, vasculitis, Sjögren's syndrome and lung involvement. IgG and monomeric IgM rheumatoid factors are associated with vasculitis in rheumatoid arthritis and IgA rheumatoid

Table 8.1 Diseases with IgM rheumatoid factor

Disease	Incidence
Rheumatoid arthritis	
Overall	70%
With nodules	99%
Sjögren's syndrome	100%
SLE	
Progressive systemic sclerosis	35%
Mixed connective tissue disease	
Other diseases	
Chronic active hepatitis and other chronic liver disorders	
Fibrosing alveolitis	
Paraproteinaemias	
Chronic infections	
Subacute bacterial endocarditis	
Pulmonary tuberculosis	
Infectious mononucleosis	
Syphilis	
Leprosy	
Others	
Elderly people	5% (low titre)
Relatives of patients with RA	

factors with primary Sjögren's syndrome, but these tests are at present of research interest and are not routinely used by clinicians.

Antinuclear antibody

A variety of antibodies to different nuclear and cytoplasmic cellular components are found in connective tissue diseases.

Fluorescent antinuclear antibody (ANA)

This is the screening test for SLE (having replaced the lupus erythematosus cell test) and is positive in at least 95% of cases. ANA is also found in other connective tissue diseases including rheumatoid arthritis (RA), progressive systemic sclerosis, mixed connective tissue disease and myositis. Various patterns of nuclear staining are seen and are associated with antibodies to different antigenic components (Table 8.2). Antibodies producing a speckled pattern are directed against 'extractable nuclear antigens' (ENA). Over twenty antinuclear and anticytoplasmic antibodies have now been identified, of which a small number have clinical significance. Disease associations for some of the

Table 8.2 Immunofluorescence patterns of antinuclear staining and the antibody associations

Pattern	Antigen
Homogeneous	Histones
Rim	Native DNA
Speckled	Non-histone proteins, Ro, La, Sm, ribonucleoproteins
Nucleolar	Nucleolar RNA (Sjögren's and progressive systemic sclerosis)

Table 8.3 Associations of some non-histone antigens with connective tissue diseases

Antigen	Disease association
Sm	SLE
Ro and La	SLE, Sjögren's syndrome
Nuclear ribonucleoprotein (high titre)	MCTD
Scl 70	Progressive systemic sclerosis
Centromere	CREST
RANA	RA and Sjögren's syndrome + RA

Abbreviations: MCTD = mixed connective tissue diseases (SLE, systemic sclerosis, myositis); CREST = 'Overlap' of calcinosis, Raynaud's phenomenon, esophageal dysmotility, sclerodactyly and telangectasia; RANA = Rheumatoid arthritis nuclear antigen.

soluble non-histone antigens are shown in Table 8.3. A few patients with clinical SLE have a negative ANA test. Such patients may have antibodies to ENA, such as anti-Ro (also called anti-SSA). Antibodies to ENA are detected by immuno-diffusion or electrophoresis.

Circulating antibodies to double-stranded DNA are the most specific test for SLE and in high titre are almost pathognomonic for the disease. The titre of DNA antibodies in some patients reflects disease activity and can be used to monitor response to therapy. Anti-DNA is often seen in chronic active hepatitis and rarely in Sjögren's syndrome or rheumatoid vasculitis. The DNA antibody test is not a screening test for SLE and should only be requested after the ANA test is shown to be positive. Antibodies to single stranded DNA (ssDNA) are found in various diseases but are not specific.

Lupus anticoagulant

Some patients with lupus-like disease and a history of recurrent abortions, venous or arterial thrombosis and thrombocytopenia, may have an antiphos-pholipid or anticardiolipin antibody, also called the 'lupus anticoagulant'. This antibody can be detected by the prolongation of the kaolin cephalin clotting time (KCCT) on routine testing. A mixing test is then performed with normal plasma to show the presence of an immediately acting inhibitor of coagulation. The lupus anticoagulant may give rise to a biological false positive test for syphilis owing to the cardiolipin in the Venereal Disease Reference Laboratory (VDRL) substrate. The antibody has been found in association with a variety of clinical conditions apart from SLE.

Acute phase reactants

The ESR is the most widely used test. The acute phase protein, C-reactive protein (CRP), can be a useful guide to disease activity and monitoring treatment of inflammatory rheumatic diseases. CRP levels are usually high with inflamma-tion but may be normal in SLE or Sjögren's syndrome despite active disease and even a high ESR. In such patients, intercurrent infection can cause elevation of CRP which may be of some value in the assessment of SLE with fever.

Complement

Since the components of complement are acute phase reactants, raised complement levels are found in many inflammatory rheumatic diseases. Synovial fluid complement levels are low in rheumatoid arthritis and high in Reiter's syndrome, but these are of little diagnostic value. Blood C_3 and C_4 levels are low in lupus nephropathy owing to consumption during the disease process.

The haemolytic activity of complement CH_{50} can be useful in the management of SLE, where a falling level indicates worsening disease.

Immune complexes

Immune complexes (IC) are found at some stage in most connective tissue diseases. The detection of IC depends on their structural and functional characteristics and many assays are available which may not give concordant results in the same patient. The most widely used test for IC is the C1q, binding method. At present, IC are a rather non-specific test, like the ESR, and clinical decisions are not often made on the results of assays, but this may change in the future.

Polyclonal serum cryoglobulin precipitates are found in RA, particularly in association with vasculitis, Sjögren's or Felty's syndromes, and their demonstration is by a simple and cheap test. The blood sample must be transported to the laboratory, allowed to clot and separated, all at 37°C, before cooling to 4°C for 72 h during the test.

Tissue typing antigens

The most frequently requested antigen is the Class I* HLA B27. A positive result can contribute to the diagnosis in a patient who has 'reactive' arthritis (present in 60%) or early ankylosing spondylitis (over 95%), but there is no value in requesting the test when the diagnosis is obvious. The antigen is found in 7% of the general population and may be a co-incidental finding (only 5% of B27-positive people develop spondylitis).

Radiological investigations

General

Radiological investigation of clinically affected joints is an important assessment in many rheumatic conditions. There is little point in taking an X-ray of soft tissue injuries or inflammatory arthritis where the history is short (less than 4 months) and when there are no clinical signs—the exceptions being chondrocalcinosis and septic arthritis. Current X-rays are important when considering a patient for orthopaedic or plastic surgery. A routine chest X-ray is usually performed. Pulmonary carcinoma, tuberculosis and sarcoidosis are examples of disease which may result in a patient presenting with rheumatic symptoms. Respiratory and cardiovascular complications can occur as part of a systemic disease process in rheumatoid arthritis, seronegative arthritis and other connective tissue diseases.

---

* Class I antigens are glycoproteins found on the surface of most nucleated cells. Class II antigens are restricted to certain cells within the immune system.

Rheumatoid arthritis

1 The earliest changes are likely to be seen in the feet, hands and wrists. These are easy to radiograph and usually only require one projection.

2 Look for soft tissue swelling, peri-articular osteoporosis and marginal erosions (junction of the synovium with articular cartilage).

3 Later changes include further loss of joint space, more destructive, erosive damage; subluxation or dislocation; ankylosis (usually in the wrist) and secondary degenerative changes.

4 Serial X-rays at extended intervals (6 months or 1 year) provide evidence of disease progression. The progression is usually uniform and so it is not necessary to take X-rays of all the joints each time.

5 Cervical spine; instability of the cervical spine can be demonstrated by a single lateral X-ray with the neck in flexion. The distance between the front surface of the odontoid peg (axis) and anterior arch of the atlas should be less than 3–4 mm. Subluxation may occur at other levels in the cervical spine. Unrecognized subluxation can result in damage to the spinal cord, particularly during anaesthesia manoeuvres.

6 The chest X-ray may show evidence of pleural effusion, fibrosing alveolitis or nodules.

Osteoarthritis

Clinical examination may be sufficient to make a confident diagnosis but X-rays are often taken. Characteristic changes are: joint space narrowing due to thinning of the cartilage, subchondral sclerosis, osteophyte formation and subchondral cysts. To assess the true degree of cartilage loss and joint space narrowing in the knee, a weight-bearing view should be taken. 'Skyline' angled views are required to see the patellofemoral joint. Sometimes erosive appearances due to osteoarthritis in the distal interphalangeal (DIP) and proximal interphalangeal (PIP) finger joints may mimic inflammatory arthritis, particularly that associated with psoriasis.

Seronegative arthritis

Sacro-iliitis

In a young adult patient with early-morning low-back stiffness and pain, an X-ray may show sacro-iliitis. To outline sacro-iliac (SI) joints, which involves a substantial dose of the radiation, the X-ray beam is angled appropriately, although an antero-posterior view of the pelvis will show the SI regions obliquely. The availability of B27 antigen testing in larger centres assists with the clinical diagnosis of early ankylosing spondylitis when radiological signs are equivocal.

More established radiological changes of sacro-iliitis, which are usually bilateral, include sclerosis of the ilium and sacrum on either side of the joint, haziness and, later, erosions of the joint margins followed by narrowing of the joint space with eventual sclerosis and a 'ghost' joint.

Ankylosing spondylitis

As the disease extends up the spine from the SI joints, features such as squaring of the lumbar vertebral bodies and calcification of annulus fibrosus and interspinous ligaments are seen.

Once the diagnosis of ankylosing spondylitis is established, then X-rays are mainly used to assess peripheral arthritis and axial disease is followed using clinical measurements.

Reiter's syndrome, psoriasis and enteropathic arthritis

There is little point in taking X-rays of patients during the early stages of Reiter's syndrome. If the disease becomes protracted or recurrent, changes similar to rheumatoid arthritis may occur, but with a different distribution. Juxta-articular osteoporosis may be seen, or joint space narrowing and erosive damage affecting the metatarsophalangeal (MTP) joints asymmetrically, the interphalangeal (IP) joint of the hallux and the os calcis at the insertion of the Achilles tendon. Other changes include fluffy peri-osteal new bone formations, affecting bone next to involved joints (also seen in psoriatic arthritis), calcaneal spurs, sacro-iliitis and spondylitis. The hands are rarely involved.

Psoriatic arthritis changes on X-ray may be similar to rheumatoid disease, although with less juxta-articular osteoporosis and more bony ankylosis. Sacro-iliitis and spondylitis can occur, also a destructive form of erosion with bone resorption leading to the 'pencil-in-cup' appearance of psoriatic arthritis mutilans.

The arthropathies associated with inflammatory bowel disease are not usually erosive nor do they show any radiological changes.

Other radiological tests

Arthrography

Most commonly performed in the knee. Injection of contrast medium into the synovial cavity can demonstrate a posterior capsular protrusion or Baker's cyst. If this ruptures, clinical manifestations simulating a deep venous thrombosis (DVT) may present, but the radiopaque dye will be seen extravasated into the calf. Arthrography of the knee can also allow conditions such as menisceal tears, pigmented villonodular synovitis and synovial chondromatosis to be excluded.

Computerized tomographic scanning

The CT scan can produce excellent resolution of both bony structures and soft tissues. This may be of particular value in the evaluation of back pain. Vertebral bodies can be well-visualized, showing evidence of trauma, arthritis or infiltrative disease. Back pain due to lesions on the posterior abdominal wall may be diagnosed and anatomical areas which are difficult to demonstrate by conventional means can be visualized, such as the thoracic inlet, SI joints, and Achilles tendons. Magnetic resonance imaging (MRI) gives better definition than CT scans and will be increasingly valuable in larger centres.

Diagnostic ultrasound

This can be used to evaluate mass lesions in the calf, e.g. distinguishing Baker's cyst from joint rupture or venous thrombosis.

Angiography

Angiograms of renal or mesenteric vessels may be contributory to the diagnosis of polyarteritis nodosa (PAN) with multiple small aneurysms in up to 80% of cases; the investigation can be more useful than 'blind' muscle biopsy.

Radioisotope scanning

Using bone-seeking isotopes, such as technetium diphosphonate, the radioactivity over an inflamed joint can be measured. The technique provides a useful means of detecting secondary malignant deposits or infections in bone, particularly the spine. Paget's disease, osteoid osteoma and established avascular necrosis show up brightly on the scan. Joint imaging may be used to demonstrate pathology in joints not easily seen on radiographs, such as rheumatoid disease in the temporomandibular joint or inflammation of the costochondral junctions.

Autologous indium-labelled leucocyte preparations can be used specifically to localize and detect septic joints, particularly in the hips. The technique is both highly sensitive and specific. Gallium-67 localizes into areas of increased metabolic activity, such as sarcoid granulomata.

Thermography

Skin temperature reflects underlying vascularity and a thermographic map can be made to document either increased blood flow associated with inflammation or impaired perfusion, as with Raynaud's phenomenon.

Synovial investigation—fluid, arthroscopy and biopsy

Synovial fluid is an ultrafiltrate of plasma, also containing hyaluronate secreted by synovial cells. The normal protein concentration is between $10-30\,\mathrm{g\,l^{-1}}$, most of which is albumin with small amounts of fibrinogen and globulin. Small molecular weight substances cross the synovium freely and are present with equal concentration in plasma and synovial fluid.

The principal diagnostic value of synovial fluid examination is to detect crystals or infection.

Aspiration

The knee is the most frequently and easily aspirated joint. Using an aseptic technique, with the patient lying down and the quadriceps muscle relaxed, the knee joint is entered with a 21 gauge needle, usually under the medial lower edge of the patella. Local anaesthetic is unnecessary unless there may be difficulty locating the joint space. Synovial fluid is withdrawn and placed in appropriate containers for microscopy and bacteriology (sterile) and sometimes biochemical analysis (plain or heparinized). A sample may be sent in EDTA or a heparinized container for cell counts.

Table 8.4 Analysis of synovial fluid

Type	Colour	Clarity	Viscosity	Cell count mm^{-3}
Normal	Colourless/ Straw	Clear	High	<200 <25% polymorphs
Non-inflammatory	Straw/yellow	Clear	High	200–2000 <25% polymorphs
Inflammatory	Yellow	Translucent/ opaque	Low	3000–75000 >50% polymorphs
Septic	Variable	Opque/turbid	Variable	>100 000 usually >90% polymorphs

Appearance

Normal fluid, present in only very small amounts, is colourless, clear, viscous and does not clot. Inflammatory changes result in cloudy, less viscous fluid which clots on standing due to the raised fibrinogen content. Osteoarthritis is associated with clear viscous synovial fluid whilst in a septic arthritis it is thin and cloudy/purulent. Haemarthrosis may indicate trauma, haemophilia or villonodular synovitis. A summary of synovial fluid analysis is shown in Table 8.4.

Microscopy of synovial fluid

A white blood cell count (WBC) is carried out on an anticoagulated sample. Normal synovial fluid contains fewer than 200 wbc mm^{-3}, lymphocytes being predominant. If infection is considered, a Gram stain should be performed to look for organisms.

Crystals are sought in a fresh, non-anticoagulated specimen. If a clot has formed, this should also be examined because it may enmesh crystals. A polarizing microscope is used and with a first-order compensator, it is possible to distinguish urate and pyrophosphate crystals by their optical characteristics. Urate crystals are needle-shaped, weakly negatively birefringent and, when the long axis is parallel to the slow component of the compensator, the crystals appear yellow and then blue when at right angles. Pyrophosphate crystals are more brick-shaped, positively birefringent and behave the opposite way to urate with the first-order compensator. Calcium hydroxyapatite crystals can cause acute calcific peri-arthritis and may be found in synovial fluid during episodes of synovitis in osteoarthritis. The crystals are too small to be seen on light microscopy unless present as aggregates.

If more definitive identification of crystals is required, then X-ray diffraction or electron probe analysis may be used.

Arthroscopy

The main use of arthroscopy is for direct examination of the knee joint. Under local anaesthetic a limited view is obtained, but with general anaesthesia a full examination can be made to assess the state of the menisci and cruciate ligaments, seeking loose bodies, obtaining synovial biopsies and looking for causes of unexplained pain.

Synovial biopsy

Synovium may be obtained by blind needle biopsy, through an arthroscope or at open surgery. The Parker–Pearson needle is most often used and small pieces of tissue obtained for histology, microbiological culture or crystal examination. Immunofluorescent and electron microscopy can be studied. Monoarthritis may be an indication, and particularly if TB is suspected, but negative biopsy does not exclude this diagnosis.

Other biopsies

Skin

Skin histology can be diagnostic, as in sarcoidosis or non-specific, as in many forms of vasculitis. The lupus band test is sometimes performed, looking for the deposition of immunoglobulin and complement at the dermal–epidermal junction in non-involved skin. The test is not always positive in lupus, nor specific for that disease.

Temporal artery

The temporal artery is biopsied in a patient who may have giant cell arteritis. A 2 cm specimen length is obtained if possible because pathological involvement is not continuous and so, sampling error can occur.

Muscle

The diagnosis of polymyositis includes muscle biopsy, electromyography (EMG) and creatine kinase (CK) enzyme estimation. The muscle biopsy may be done with a needle, usually into the quadriceps muscle or 'open' in theatre. The muscle tissue should be prepared specially by the histology staff, particularly if histochemical staining is being done. EMG is performed on non-biopsied muscle. 'Blind' needle muscle biopsy, usually from a quadriceps muscle, may be performed to look for histological evidence of polyarteritis nodosa.

Summary of diagnostic approach

The management of rheumatic symptoms at the time of presentation is summarized in Fig. 8.1.

Once a diagnosis is made, even if the problem remains imprecise, it is useful to consider next the underlying pathological process. Typical examples are shown in Table 8.5.

The investigation sequence of rheumatic disease is outlined below. Clearly, such investigations will not always be required, and the degree of investigation will vary according to the individual circumstance.

Investigation of rheumatic disease

Careful history and examination.
1 *First stage investigations.* As appropriate:
   (a) Full blood count, ESR/viscosity.
   (b) Biochemistry—electrolytes, liver function, urate.
   (c) Immunology—RA latex, ANA.

(d) Viral serology.

(e) Radiology. Request most involved joints, but only if abnormality likely, i.e. not acute onset or soft tissue. Chest X-ray.

(f) Aspirate synovial fluid for appearance, consistency, bacteriology or crystals (may be the last chance for gout).

2 *Second stage investigations* may be indicated initially or at follow-up:

(a) Blood tests for: further immunology, DNA binding, ENA, complement, immune complexes, B_{27} antigen, follow-up viral titres, biochemistry, e.g. CK enzyme.

(b) Radiology. Special views, e.g. SI joints, IVU or angiography.

(c) Radioisotope scanning or thermography.

3 *Third stage investigations:*

(a) Arthroscopy.

(b) Biopsies of synovium, skin, temporal artery or muscle.

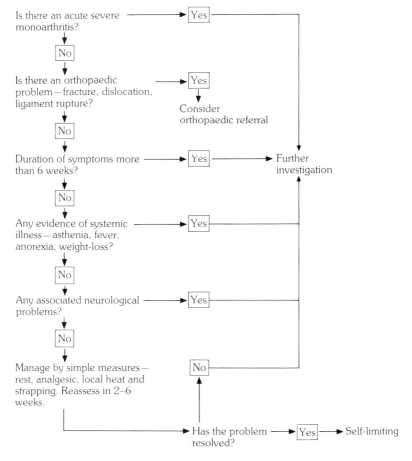

Fig. 8.1 Algorithm for the management of a rheumatic patient at the point of presentation.

Table 8.5 Main pathological categories of rheumatic diseases

Pathological process	Disease	Initial tests
Synovitis	Rheumatoid arthritis	RA latex, ESR, full blood count
Degeneration of cartilage	Osteoarthritis	X-ray relevant joints
Enthesopathy	Ankylosing spondylitis	X-ray SI joints, B_{27} antigen
Local enthesopathy	Tennis *or* golfer's elbow	Nil *or* local X-rays
Crystal synovitis	Gout *or* pseudogout	Aspiration *and* microscopic crystal detection
Joint infection	Staphylococcal septic arthritis	Aspiration *and* microbiology
Myositis or myopathy	Polymyositis	Serum creatine kinase, muscle biopsy (EMG)
Non-specific	Minor trauma, fibrositis	Nil *or* ESR *and* full blood count

Chapter 9
Obstetrics and Gynaecology

OBSTETRICS

Introduction

Pregnancy is a state of health, but most pregnant women in this country have multiple screening investigations performed to identify individuals who have, or are at risk of, particular complications. Much of this chapter is devoted to the further investigation of women identified as being at risk, by such screening.

Specific investigations

Routine tests at first antenatal clinic in early pregnancy

These are shown in Table 9.1.

In addition the maternal serum alpha-fetoprotein is checked at 16–18 weeks and many centres now perform ultrasound scans for confirmation of menstrual dates and to exclude multiple pregnancy and fetal abnormality.

Pregnancy tests

The most commonly used pregnancy tests are based on the principle of latex agglutination inhibition. This test detects the presence of human chorionic gonadotropin (HCG) in the urine.

More recently, enzyme-linked immunosorbent assays (ELISA) are becoming more popular. These are highly specific for HCG and can give a reliable positive test about 2 weeks after ovulation.

Haemoglobin

This should be within the normal range at first visit but often falls to a nadir around 30 weeks, owing largely to a dilutional effect of the physiological expansion in plasma volume. Haemoglobin (Hb) is checked in all women at their first visit, and again at about 32 weeks gestation. Women at increased risk of

Table 9.1 Routine tests at first antenatal clinic in early pregnancy

Pregnancy test (for confirmation of pregnancy)
Blood group and antibody screen
VDRL/TPHA
Rubella antibodies
MSU
Cervical smear (if not checked within the previous 3 years)

Abbreviations: VDRL = Venereal Disease Research Laboratory test; TPHA = *Treponema pallidum* haemagglutination assay; MSU = mid-stream urine specimen.

anaemia in pregnancy (e.g. those with multiple pregnancies or who have had recurrent vaginal bleeding) require more frequent checks. A low Hb (<10 g dl^{-1}) requires investigation.

Blood group and antibody screen

All women have their blood group identified early in pregnancy, primarily to identify those who are Rhesus (D) antigen negative (antigens C and E are less important in stimulating antibody formation) or who already have antibodies. This minority group of RhD – ve (approximately 13% of the British population) are at risk of being exposed to Rhesus antigen (D) if they carry a fetus which is Rhesus (D) positive and if any fetomaternal transfusion occurs. Parturition is the time of particular risk of fetomaternal transfusion, although miscarriage, antepartum bleeding or amniocentesis can also sensitize the mother to fetal blood cells. Rhesus negative mothers have further antibody screening at about 26 and 34 weeks gestation.

The *Kleihauer test* is a means of detecting *fetal* cells in the maternal circulation, and depends on the differing response of adult and fetal red blood cells when exposed to alkaline buffer.

VDRL/TPHA

False positive tests for syphilis are now six times more common than true positives. A positive TPHA is usually repeated and syphilitic infection confirmed by more specific tests, such as the fluorescent treponemal antibody-absorption test (FTA-ABS) or the *Treponema pallidum* immobilization test (TPI). Nevertheless, biological false positives may occur with these tests in women with systemic lupus erythematosus (SLE) which causes chronic biological false positive FTA-ABS or TPI owing to the presence of anti-D DNA antibody.

Rubella antibodies

Women who have no immunity are usually advised to have the vaccine postnatally. Women who have antibodies at booking require no further investigation during that pregnancy but should be rechecked in each subsequent pregnancy as immunity derived from vaccination as a child does not always confer life-long protection and antibody titres can wane. Women who give a history of recent exposure to rubella in the first trimester of pregnancy and who are not known to be immune, have two blood samples taken 2 weeks apart. If the antibody titre rises sharply between the two samples this is strongly suggestive of recent infection. Most laboratories can now offer IgM titres. Since IgM is the earliest response to first infection, a high IgM titre confirms that the patient was not previously immune.

Mid-stream urine specimen

A mid-stream urine specimen (MSU) is taken at the first visit to detect asymptomatic bacteruria, which denotes the risk of developing acute pyelonephritis later in pregnancy. Confirmed urinary tract infection necessitates antibiotic sensitivity testing.

Women who have several proven urinary infections during their pregnancy should undergo investigation of their renal tract once they have delivered.

Serum alpha-fetoprotein (AFP)

This is used as a screening test for fetal neural tube defects. See Tables 9.2 and 9.3.

Table 9.2 Causes of high AFP

Wrong dates
Twins
Bleeding—recent threatened abortion
Neural tube defects—anencephaly and open spina bifida (Meningomyeloceles) (marked elevation)
Any other breech of the fetal surface, e.g. exomphalos/omphalocele/ectopia/vesica
Recent intra-uterine fetal death

Table 9.3 Causes of Low AFP

Wrong dates
Missed abortion
Down's syndrome fetus. Sensitivity of the test is increased when carried out in conjunction with HCG levels

Ultrasound

Pre-conception

Ovaries can be visualized, developing follicles observed. Follicles can even be punctured transabdominally or transvesically if oocytes are required to be harvested for *in vitro* fertilization.

Early pregnancy

1 6 weeks: an intra-uterine sac is visible. This is valuable information where tubal pregnancy is suspected.

2 8–10 weeks: the gestation sac and fetus are visible. Gestation can be assessed by measuring crown–rump length (CRL) The fetal heart movements are clearly seen.

Placental site is identifiable if chorion villous biopsy is being considered.

3 12 weeks: most fetal parts identifiable and some gross abnormalities detected, e.g. anencephaly, large exomphalos.

4 16 weeks: a sufficiently large pool of fluid can generally be found to permit amniocentesis.

5 16–20 weeks: this period gives the most accurate assessment of gestational age. Fetal parts are sufficiently large for comment on anatomical normality. The fetal spine, abdomen and head can be visualized.

6 30–40 weeks: if intra-uterine growth retardation is suspected, a scan at this stage can measure the fetal size. Biparietal diameter (BPD) is not a good reflection of intra-uterine growth as even fetuses that are failing to thrive *in utero* tend to have near normal head growth. The 'head-sparing' effect, which may be a reflection of the fetal circulation which favours organs supplied by the arch of the aorta, led to a number of other measurements being used to assess fetal weight. Fetal trunk area (FTA) can be calculated from the abdominal circumference at the fixed level of the umbilical cord to detect the abdominal size, but this varies considerably with the degree of fetal flexion. For this reason, trunk area × crown–rump length is often used instead: over 90% of growth-retarded fetuses can be correctly identified at 34 weeks gestation, provided that there was an earlier scan to confirm gestational age.

Placental site can be identified readily at this stage of pregnancy.

Investigations for fetal abnormality

Apart from maternal alpha-fetoprotein and ultrasound scanning, further investigations are available to identify specific fetal abnormalities in women at particular risk.

Amniocentesis

A sample of amniotic fluid is removed from the uterus of the pregnant woman at 16 weeks gestation. The subsequent miscarriage risk is about 1%. The patient must be clear about the limitations of the test and the action that can be taken once the results are known.

Only certain fetal abnormalities can be diagnosed and false, negative results, although uncommon, do occur.

The investigation may not produce any result if the amniotic fetal desquamated cells fail to grow in tissue cultures.

Indications for amniocentesis

The most common indications are outlined below.

Chromosomal analysis

Maternal age: over the age of 37 years, the risk of a woman with no family history of Down's syndrome conceiving a child with this condition rises to 1%. Over 40 years of age it is 2% and this rises to 4% in women over 44 years. Younger women are often offered the investigation if they have had a previously affected infant.

Fetal sexing: women who have given birth to male infants suffering from an X-linked recessive-type genetic disorder frequently request amniocentesis.

Single gene defects: many diseases are caused by single gene defects, either X-linked recessive conditions affecting male offspring or autosomal recessives affecting both sexes. Only a few of these disorders can yet be predicted by amniocentesis and the diagnosis is usually less definite than with chromosomal abnormalities. To diagnose a single gene defect it is usually necessary to look for its expression, as with abnormal metabolic products.

Chorion villous biopsy

At about 6–8 weeks from the last menstrual period the placental site becomes apparent on ultrasound scan as the trophoblast rapidly proliferates in one area and regresses in others. Chorion villi abound here.

The procedure is usually performed between 9 and 11 weeks and the cytogeneticist usually requires 10 mg of good quality *branching* villi.

The risk of miscarriage following the procedure is about 2% above the background incidence at this point in gestation, but this risk increases with the number of attempts and is higher in centres with less experience of the technique.

The chorionic villi can be grown in tissue cultures for karyotyping. Gene probes are currently available for some gene defects.

Fetoscopy

Fetoscopy is an invasive investigative technique, whereby the developing fetus is visualized *in utero* by passing a thin fibreoptic endoscope transabdominally into the uterus.

Investigation of fetal health

There are basically two main questions obstetricians want answered in later pregnancy (after 28 weeks): (i) Is the fetus growing (getting enough nutrients)? (ii) Is the baby receiving enough oxygen?

Both questions relate to the quality of placental function; the first to chronic failure and the second concerned with more acute inadequacy.

1 Is the fetus growing?

(a) **Palpation of the uterine fundus** correctly predicts only 50% of low birth-weight babies.

(b) **Ultrasound scanning** has largely replaced all previous investigations for fetal growth.

(c) **Biochemical investigation of fetal growth.** The two most commonly performed investigations were assays of the placental steroid, oestriol, and of the placental protein, human placenta lactogen (HPL), but these have now been largely replaced by ultrasound scanning.

2 Is the fetus getting enough oxygen? The placenta's ability to transfer nutrients from the maternal to the fetal circulation is a major determinant of fetal growth, but its ability to transfer oxygen is vital to fetal survival. The question is relatively easy to answer when the mother is in *labour* with *ruptured membranes* and a sample of fetal scalp capillary blood can be analysed, but during the antenatal period prior to this, reliance must must be placed on less direct measurements which are known to reflect fetal oxygenation to a greater or lesser degree.

Cardiotocography. This is one of the most commonly used indirect investigations of fetal oxygenation. It involves recording the fetal heart rate and its variation, usually over at least 20–30 min. Movement of the heart valves, by a Doppler effect, causes a change in observed frequency of the ultrasound beam reflected from the heart back to the transducer and this is electronically converted into a printout tracing of fetal heart rate.

The fetal heart rate of a full-term fetus should be between 120 and 160 beats per min. There is normally a degree of variability between the rate from one 5-second period to the next, rather than an absolutely regular interval from one beat to the next.

In addition, the fetal heart usually responds to uterine contractions or fetal movements by accelerating for a minute or two before returning to the baseline rate.

Several patterns of fetal heart rate seen on cardiotocography are known to be ominous and associated with poor outcome.

In labour, measurement of the fetal heart rate is much simpler because once the membranes are ruptured, a fetal scalp electrode can be applied.

Fetal blood sampling. Measuring the fetal heart rate can give a guide to the fetal condition, but only about 50% of fetuses with ominous features on cardiotocography have low oxygen tensions in cord blood at birth or are born in poor condition. A more direct measure of poor fetal oxygenation can be obtained by scalp blood sampling after rupture of the membranes.

GYNAECOLOGY

Introduction

Investigation of menstrual disorders is one of the commonest reasons for gynaecological referral. There are broadly three main groups of complaints: amenorrhoea; heavy or heavy and prolonged bleeding (menorrhagia); and post-menopausal bleeding. Amenorrhoea is said to be primary if periods have not commenced by the age of 16 years and secondary where regular menses have occurred but ceased. Menorrhagia involves a subjective observation by the patient that her periods are heavier and more prolonged than they were previously. Post-menopausal bleeding always prompts consideration of endometrial carcinoma and thus, usually merits investigation.

The three other main subdivisions of gynaecological practice are: oncology, infertility; and urodynamics.

Cervical cancer is a common condition which may be prevented by screening for premalignant change. Unfortunately, ovarian cancer tends to present when relatively advanced.

Since normally fertile couples may take a variable time to achieve pregnancy, it is important to establish a time by which pregnancy might be expected to occur in order to define infertility. About 90% of couples have achieved a pregnancy after 1 year of normal intercourse without contraception. Of the remaining 10% some may achieve pregnancy without medical intervention but many will have an identifiable cause for their failure to conceive.

The majority of women attending gynaecological out-patient clinics on account of incontinence complain of loss of urinary control on bending or coughing, with no prior sensation of desire to micturate, this is defined as stress incontinence. It is normally associated with urethral sphincter weakness and is considered potentially curable by surgery. The second most common cause is detrusor instability in which the bladder muscle contracts in an uninhibited fashion, causing the intravesical pressure to exceed the urethral pressure and presenting as urge incontinence. These patients will not be helped by surgery.

Specific investigations

Oncology

There is only one screening investigation in widespread gynaecological use— exfoliative cervical cytology by scraping the surface of the cervix with a disposable wooden spatula to detect asymptomatic pre-invasive disease of the cervix.

Interpretation

Cervical cytology is a *screening* procedure designed to detect which women may have asymptomatic pre-invasive disease of the cervical epithelium at a stage when it is easily treated. It is *not* a *diagnostic* investigation. The cytologist can only tell whether or not there is a dyskaryosis and thus decide which women might benefit from further investigation. The degree of dyskaryosis on *cytology* correlates poorly with the underlying *histology* on subsequent biopsy, but it can give a guide to the likely findings.

Further investigation of abnormal smears

The cervix can be visualized with the colposcope, a binocular microscope usually offering magnification of $\times 10 - \times 30$. Acetic acid staining produces a characteristic change in the colour of the cervix where areas of epithelium are dysplastic, usually producing an opaque white appearance. Other atypical appearances include mosaic or punctate vascular patterns. The most abnormal-looking area of the cervix should reveal the most dysplastic area within the epithelium and sometimes two or three punch biopsies are taken. These biopsies are only about 2 mm across, i.e. much smaller than a cone biopsy. The procedure is carried out without anaesthesia as an out-patient. Bleeding is minimal.

Women who fall into the group where the whole epithelium cannot be seen are classed as having unsatisfactory colposcopies and require cone biopsy. This problem mainly arises in older women. A second group of women who often require cone biopsy are those in whom microinvasive disease is suspected on colposcopy.

Endometrial carcinoma

There is no screening programme for this disease which fortunately tends to present early, usually in post-menopausal women with vaginal bleeding.

Dilatation and curettage

This is one of the most commonly performed diagnostic investigations. Fractional curettage offers the most accurate staging of tumour spread as the endocervix is curetted separately to determine whether tumour has spread to the endocervix, which changes the staging of the carcinoma and the prognosis.

Vabra curettage

The slimness of the curette (which is attached to a small vacuum pump) allows it to be inserted through an undilated cervix and thus obviates the need for general anaesthesia. However, the technique can produce only a small strip of tissue for histology.

Ovarian carcinoma

Although the incidence of ovarian carcinoma is less than cervical or endometrial carcinoma, it still heads the league table for deaths from gynaecological malignancy, largely because in the early stages the disease is asymptomatic and because there is as yet no effective screening technique available. The time of diagnosis for many patients is during laparotomy, by which time the disease is often already advanced and there is often little point in pre-operative investigation apart from a chest X-ray. Many oncologists favour sampling the pelvic and para-aortic lymph nodes for signs of lymphatic invasion.

Blood tumour markers

Carcinoplacental antigens

These are ectopically produced antigens which are normally present only in the placenta, but can be found in the blood after malignant transformation of certain tissues.

Placental alkaline phosphatase. These phosphatases are biochemically distinct from those found in bone, intestine, kidney and liver. The Regan isoenzyme is elevated in the majority of patients with ovarian carcinoma and to a lesser degree in many other malignancies.

Placental hormones. Human chorionic gonadotrophin is normally elevated only during pregnancy. It has proved an ideal tumour marker for hydatidiform mole and choriocarcinoma in that it is consistently present in all such tumours; its level quantitatively correlates with the tumour bulk, is reduced by successful chemotherapy and increases if recurrence occurs.

Human placental lactogen is elevated in 76% of patients with epithelial ovarian carcinomas but is more specific for germ cell ovarian tumours containing ectopic trophoblastic tissue.

Tumour associated antigens

These are glycoproteins that are present on the cell surface of ovarian cancer cells, but are absent from benign ovarian tissue. These ovarian cancer-associated antigens are assumed to arise during the malignant transformation process. One of these, ovarian carcinoma-associated antigen (OCAA), has been found in 70% of patients with ovarian carcinoma. Unfortunately, not only does this investigation miss over a quarter of the women with ovarian carcinoma but it has also been found that the correlation between clinical course and the rise and fall in OCAA levels is very poor.

Fetal antigens
These are mainly glycoproteins that are present in the fetus during early pregnancy but should have disappeared shortly after birth. When certain malignancies develop they reappear on the surface membranes of the tumour cells.

Alpha-fetoprotein (AFP). This is a fetal antigen produced in the human liver and yolk sac of the placenta in the first two trimesters. It is a specific tumour marker for the rare endodermal sinus tumours of the ovary, embryonal carcinoma of the ovary and ovarian teratomas. It is *not* elevated in the common epithelial ovarian carcinomas. It is an almost perfect tumour marker for endodermal sinus tumour of the ovary as it is present in the majority of such tumours, decreases in response to therapy and increases with recurrence.

Carcinoembryoma antigen, beta-oncofetoprotein and fetal ferritin. These have all been found in ovarian carcinoma, but are not specific for this condition.
    Unlike tumour-associated antigens, fetal antigens are minimally antigenic and can occur in various tumours as well as in normal tissues.

Infertility

Causes
In approximately 40% of cases a female factor is responsible, in 40% a male factor is responsible and in 10% both partners have a contributing cause. In 10% of cases infertility is unexplained and both partners appear fertile on investigation.

Male factors
There are two main factors to consider: (i) ability to have normal intercourse; and (ii) quality of semen.

Ability to have normal intercourse
Physical problems include: spina bifida, paraplegia, hypospadias. Psychological problems include: impotence, premature ejaculation. The problem will become apparent on history and physical examination.

Quality of semen
Semen varies in quantity and quality between individuals and in the same individual at different times. It is recommended that at least three seminal specimens are analysed. Minimum criteria for fertility are given in Table 9.4. It is being increasingly recognized that many men appear to have normal fertility

Table 9.4 Minimum criteria for fertility

Volume	>2 ml
Sperm density	>20 000 000 ml^{-1}
Sperm motility	>50%
Abnormal forms	<20%

despite relatively low sperm densities. The results of seminal analyses are dependent on the method of collection. Ideally, 3 days of abstinence from intercourse should precede the semen collection. The sample is produced by masturbation into a clean, plastic container and kept at body temperature until it is examined within a few hours.

If three such specimens yield low counts, serum follicle stimulating hormone (FSH), luteinizing hormone (LH), prolactin and testosterone should be measured. A chromosome analysis may be useful if a count less than $5\,000\,000\ ml^{-1}$ is discovered.

If sperm numbers appear adequate but *motility* is consistently low, sperm immobilizing antibodies should be looked for in serum and seminal plasma. Testicular biopsy is reserved for the few men in whom there is evidence of epididymal blockage.

Female factors

There are two important considerations: (i) ? ovulation; and (ii) ? tubal patency/function.

Ovulation

Of regularly menstruating women, 10% are not ovulating. Several investigations are in use to determine if ovulation is occurring.

Temperature chart

There is usually a slight fall in basal body temperature about the time of ovulation, followed by a sustained rise of $0.3-0.5°C$ during the luteal phase of the menstrual cycle. The temperature should be measured using a suitably accurate thermometer when the patient wakes in the morning, before any physical activity has been undertaken or anything has been consumed which might otherwise affect the temperature.

Endometrial biopsy

If a dilatation and curettage is performed 1–3 days pre-menstrually and the biopsy of endometrium obtained shows secretory changes, then ovulation is likely to have occurred during that cycle, since secretory changes in the endometrium require progesterone from an active corpus luteum.

Serum hormone assays

The most commonly performed test for 'proof' that ovulation has occurred is a single serum progesterone assay usually taken on day 21 of the cycle. When the hormone level is elevated, this is strongly indicative that ovulation has occurred. Unfortunately, the serum progesterone can be elevated by luteinization of a follicle which has not ruptured and released its ovum, so an elevated serum progesterone in the second half of the cycle only indicates that luteinization of a follicle has occurred. To be sure that release of an ovum has occurred, serial ultrasound scans are necessary.

Most infertility clinics perform several other serum hormone assays at the initial visit.

Prolactin
The serum prolactin should be measured on more than one occasion as the level can vary considerably at different times. If the level is elevated, this can cause amenorrhoea or oligomenorrhoea. A grossly elevated level is often found with pituitary microadenomas but other causes of a high serum prolactin should be excluded, especially if the level is only moderately elevated, e.g. prolactin is a hormone secreted in increased amount during times of stress.

Luteinizing hormone/follicle stimulating hormone
In polycystic ovarian disease levels of both hormones may be chronically elevated or the ratio of LH to FSH may be altered.

Thyroxine
T4 is routinely measured because there is a significant pick-up of previously undiagnosed thyroid dysfunction. Both hypothyroid and hyperthyroid states can cause ovulatory dysfunction.

Ultrasound screening
With high resolution ultrasound scanners follicles can be watched developing within the ovaries. By scanning daily during days 8–18 of a cycle, it is possible to determine whether a single follicle outgrows the others (that begin to develop in every cycle) and reaches a reasonable size (>20 mm). Follicular rupture can be assumed when such a follicle is not visible on a subsequent scan. Often a characteristic ultrasound appearance can be seen when luteinization occurs.

Tubal patency

Laparoscopy and dye insufflation
The most commonly performed investigation to establish tubal patency is laparoscopy and methylene blue dye insufflation. The pressure required to instil dye through the Fallopian tubes can be roughly gauged by the operator. The laparoscopy also permits a very good view of the pelvic organs. The Fallopian tubes are examined for signs of previous endometriosis or damage due to infection or previous surgery. The ovaries may be polycystic. A corpus luteum confirms that ovulation is occurring.

Hysterosalpingogram
This investigation involves the instillation of a radiopaque dye through the cervical os and taking one or more X-ray exposures. The investigation will:
1 Reveal whether the fallopian tubes are patent.
2 Demonstrate the site of any tubal blockage (often not possible by laparoscopy and dye instillation).
3 Delineate the intra-uterine contour to exclude an abnormality of shape, e.g. subseptate uterus (may not be apparent on external uterine appearance).

Investigation of urinary incontinence

Which women require urodynamic investigation?

Cystometry and other urodynamic investigations have been shown to be valuable in the management of women who have mixed symptoms, e.g. a bit of stress incontinence, with some urgency and perhaps nocturia. It is almost impossible to assess the underlying problem in such patients without resort to special investigations.

Cystometry

Cystometry is the measurement of bladder pressure and volume. In its simplest form cystometry involves filling the bladder via a urethral catheter attached to a central venous pressure line. The bladder is filled by a known volume of fluid and the intravesical pressure is observed on the central venous pressure gauge. It is the single most useful investigation in female urinary incontinence.

Micturating cystography

In the 1950s it was widely believed that loss of the normal posterior urethrovesical angle on coughing or straining was the main cause of genuine stress incontinence. This led to the popularity of micturating cystography.

Method. The bladder is filled with a radiopaque fluid. With the patient standing, oblique-lateral X-ray screening of the pelvis is performed. The patient is asked to cough or strain and changes in the urethrovesical angle are noted. The patient is then asked to void.

Cystoscopy

This investigation is useful if there has been any suggestion of a tumour or stone in the bladder, but it is not routinely performed in patients with incontinence. It allows a good measure of true bladder capacity, the mucosal appearance can be studied and the presence or absence of trabeculae or diverticula can be observed. The presence of neoplasia can be determined and biopsies performed for histology.

Investigation of menstrual disorders

Menorrhagia

There are two broad aetiological categories:

1 *Functional*, where the increased menstrual loss results from an identifiable organic abnormality, e.g. fibroids.

2 *Dysfunctional*, where the altered menses cannot be attributed to an obvious organic cause and are assumed to be due to endocrine disturbance.

The first question to consider is whether any investigation for this condition is required at all. For women under 40 years of age with regular menstrual cycles but heavy loss and no uterine pathology palpable at the out-patient clinic, no investigation apart from a full blood count is required. This may be true also for older women, but with increasing age many gynaecologists perform a dilatation and curettage (D & C) to exclude intra-uterine pathology, particularly endometrial carcinoma. The procedure also permits measurement of uterine size on examination under anaesthesia and measurement of uterocervical canal length. It is occasionally therapeutic as well as diagnostic on the rare occasions when an intra-uterine polyp is removed.

Post-menopausal bleeding

It is not possible to exclude endometrial carcinoma without sampling the endometrium. A D & C is therefore always advisable in post-menopausal bleeding. Apart from allowing a thorough curettage of the endometrium, a good view of the cervix and vaginal epithelium will reveal atrophic vaginitis or other local causes of bleeding.

Amenorrhoea

Investigation of primary amenorrhoea is usually required if no menstrual bleeding has occurred by the age of 16, but can be instituted earlier if there are no secondary sexual characteristics (breast-bud growth, pubic hair), especially if there are stigmata of Turner's syndrome or virilism.

There is often a history of affected 'sisters' in testicular feminization and clinical examination will reveal whether the amenorrhoea is part of a more long-standing systemic disease. Specific investigations can then be embarked upon.

Primary amenorrhoea

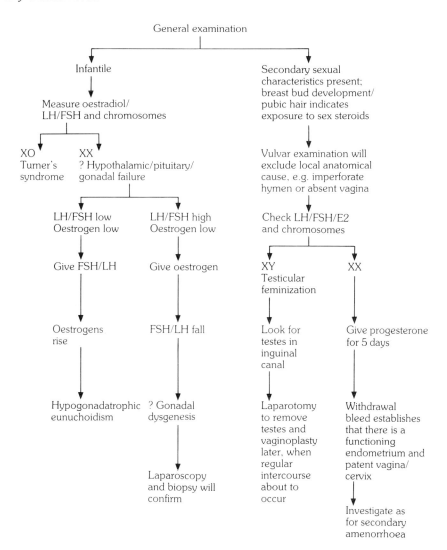

Secondary amenorrhoea/oligomenorrhoea

The fact that regular menses has occurred spontaneously in the past excludes chromosomal or congenital anatomical defects.

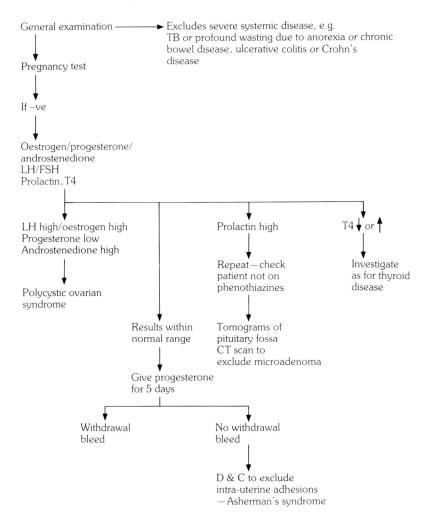

DISORDERS OF THE BREAST

Introduction

Relevant clinical investigation of patients with breast complaints is determined by three factors: (i) the sex; (ii) the age; and (iii) the complaint.

Specific investigations

Females

There is no breast disorder of sinister significance in prepubertal females and so, no specific investigations are required. Indeed, such investigations might be said

Table 9.5 Five local symptoms in adult female breasts

Pain
Lump
Nipple retraction
Nipple discharge
Skin lesions

to be meddlesome for the most commonly seen problems in these age-groups. These problems include: breast enlargement and secretion of milk in neonates, resulting from hormone overspill via the placenta; and subareolar lumps which develop in a few girls just before pubertal enlargement of the breasts commences.

There are five local symptoms which may be experienced in the adult female breast. The order of frequency in which these symptoms are likely to be reported to a doctor is shown in Table 9.5.

The clinical investigations relevant to the individual are determined on clinical grounds, the most likely cause of each symptom in a woman of the age of the particular patient presenting. A scheme summarizing these causes is given in Table 9.6.

Several investigations are technically feasible, but not all are necessarily available in every clinic. In principle, their objectives are to:
1   Provide an image of the architecture of the breast.
2   Provide material from a local site within the breast for determining morphology.

Possible investigations include:
1   *For imaging*: mammography, ultrasound, diaphonoscopy and nuclear magnetic resonance.
2   *For morphology*: fine needle aspiration cytology, disposable Trucut needle biopsy, drill biopsy and screw needle biopsy.

If after these investigations the diagnosis is still in doubt, then excision biopsy of the mass is mandatory. The clinical assessment of palpable axillary nodes is notoriously unreliable and only histological examination of the excised nodes will give a definitive answer. In the confirmed case, the so-called 'metastatic survey' should be carried out:
1   X-rays of the chest, lumbar spine and pelvis.
2   Isotope or ultrasound liver scan.

Table 9.6 Breast conditions in women of different ages

Age	Conditions
Neonatal	Hypertrophy and secretion
Prepubertal	Subareolar lump
Adolescence	Fibroadenoma
Post partum	Abscess or galactocele
Perimenopausal	Pain and cysts
Post-menopausal	Papillomata and carcinomata

3 Isotope bone scan.

However, in clinically early lesions the positive yield of these isotope investigations will be very low.

A cost-efficient and rapid method of staging breast cancer can be simply achieved by the following tests.

1 Chest X-ray for fractures, lung deposits, effusions or lymphangitis.

2 Full blood count for anaemia and film for blast cells.

3 Erythrocyte sedimentation rate (ESR), which, if raised, points to possible dissemination.

4 Blood albumin is low with liver spread; calcium and phosphate are elevated with bone secondaries.

5 Urea, creatinine, sodium, potassium and chloride as measures of renal function and to determine fitness for anaesthesia.

This simple portfolio of tests is equally useful in staging screen-detected (occult) breast cancer as symptomatic.

Males

Breast disorders are relatively uncommon in males. Prepubertal and peripubertal enlargement, lumpiness or pain in the breast in boys is never of sinister significance and requires no investigation. Persistence of gynaecomastia into late teens in males may indicate an abnormality of testicular function, possible secondary to a genetic abnormality, e.g. Klinefelter's syndrome. Serum hormones and chromosome studies will elucidate this. In men, enlargement of or lumps in breast tissue in middle or older age may be either gynaecomastia or cancer. The former may be secondary to liver disease or a side-effect of certain drugs. Fine needle aspiration cytology is a convenient and reliable method of distinguishing the benign from the malignant. Only if the cytology is equivocal is it necessary to proceed to open biopsy.

Chapter 10
Haematology

Introduction

There are very few medical disorders which do not have some effect on the blood. Similarly, primary haematological disease affects many organ systems. For these reasons haematological investigation plays an extremely important role in clinical practice.

This chapter reviews the symptoms and problems associated with haematological disease, the methods of investigation and their application in clinical management.

As in every branch of medical practice a full history and examination is of paramount importance. Thus, in a patient with anaemia, a previous history of gastric surgery, the use of non-steroidal anti-inflammatory drugs or menorrhagia constitute very important information which can obviate the need for many investigations. A dietary history can reveal the reason for haematinic deficiency; diets deficient in folic acid occur too frequently, particularly in the elderly.

General symptoms and problems

The problems with which patients present to the haematologist are outlined in Table 10.1.

Anaemia

This is the commonest manifestation of haematological disease.

Definition

Anaemia is present when the haemoglobin concentration in the circulating blood is below the normal range for the age and sex of the patient. In adults this is less than $13.0 \, \mathrm{g \, dl^{-1}}$ in males and less than $11.5 \, \mathrm{g \, dl^{-1}}$ in women. The normal range varies in childhood, being highest at the time of birth, falling to a relatively low value at 1 year of age and then gradually rising to the normal adult range after puberty.

Table 10.1 Haematological problems

Anaemia
Haemorrhagic disorder
Lymph node enlargement
Lymphomas
Myeloproliferative disorders
Myeloma
Leukaemia

179

Table 10.2 Classification of the different types of anaemia

Hypochromic microcytic anaemia
    Iron deficiency anaemia
    Thalassaemia

Normochromic normocytic anaemia
    Anaemia of chronic inflammatory disorders[*]
    Haemolytic anaemia, e.g.
        Autoimmune haemolytic anaemia
        Spherocytosis
        Glucose-6-phosphate dehydrogenase deficiency

Macrocytic anaemia
    Normoblastic macrocytic anaemia, e.g.
        Chronic liver disease
        Hypothyroidism
        Marrow aplasia *or* infiltration
    Megaloblastic macrocytic anaemia, e.g.
        Vitamin B_{12} deficiency
        Folate deficiency

[*] May be hypochromic.

Types of anaemia

The different types of anaemia are given in Table 10.2.

Symptoms of anaemia

Patients with anaemia present with two sets of symptoms; those referrable to the anaemia and those due to the underlying disease with which the anaemia is associated. Common symptoms of anaemia are given in Table 10.3.

These symptoms reflect the low haemoglobin concentration. Other features such as koilonychia, angular stomatitis or cheilitis may be associated with specific haematinic deficiencies such as iron, folate and vitamin B_{12}. Other symptoms point to the reason for the anaemia. Thus, a patient who is suffering from iron deficiency on account of gastro-intestinal blood loss may complain of epigastric pain, particularly after meals or at night. The patient with a colonic carcinoma may have noticed an alteration of bowel habit. There will usually be features of systemic disease in those patients with anaemia of inflammatory disorder.

Haemorrhagic disorders

Haemorrhagic disorders reflect defects in the platelets, blood vessels or coagulation factors.

Table 10.3 Common symptoms of anaemia

Tiredness
General muscular weakness
Breathlessness on exertion
Palpitations
Angina, claudication in a patient with vascular disease
Mental confusion and impairment of cerebral function in an elderly patient with cerebrovascular disease

Bleeding due to abnormalities of platelets or blood vessels usually occurs in the skin (petechiae and ecchymoses) and from the mucous membranes; gums, nose and gastro-intestinal tract. The usual presentation in coagulation factor deficiency is bleeding into the muscles and joints causing deep haematomas and haemarthrosis, excessive and prolonged bleeding after trauma, which may be trivial and unnoticed, and excessive bleeding after surgery, including dental extractions. Also, the pattern of bleeding after trauma is different. When haemorrhage is due to platelet or vascular defect, it occurs immediately after trauma and it may be stopped permanently by pressure on the bleeding site. When it is due to coagulation factor deficiency, haemorrhage may be delayed for several hours after trauma, and when it occurs pressure on the bleeding site has only a temporary effect and bleeding frequently restarts on removal of the pressure.

There may be a family history of bleeding disorder in patients with haemophilia; the history may also suggest vitamin C deficiency in patients with scurvy and reveal drugs which can cause thrombocytopenia (Table 10.4).

Table 10.4 Drugs which may cause thrombocytopenia

Sulphonamides
Thiazide diuretics
Quinine
Phenylbutazone
Chlorpropamide
Heparin
Gold salts

Vascular purpura is not usually very severe and is often confined to bleeding into the skin—petechiae and ecchymoses. Examples include senile purpura, ecchymoses in Cushing's syndrome and with corticosteroid therapy. Henoch–Schönlein disease may follow infection. Meningococcal septicaemia also produces a purpuric rash. Hereditary haemorrhagic telangiectasia is a rare condition which leads to bleeding from telangiectatic vessels in the gastrointestinal tract. Ehlers–Danlos disease is another rare condition associated with increased fragility of the blood vessels.

Thrombocytopenia may occur as part of another disease process, as in systemic lupus erythematosus (SLE) or acute leukaemia, or it may be induced by drug therapy. Some patients have autoimmune thrombocytopenia.

Lymphadenopathy

Enlargement of lymph nodes, with or without splenomegaly, occurs in a large variety of disorders differing widely in cause and prognosis. A lymph node greater than 1 cm in size should always be regarded as pathological. The main causes of lymph node enlargement are given in Table 10.5.

Polycythaemia

The possibility of polycythaemia may be suggested by several clinical observations. Generalized itching is a prominent symptom, thrombotic complications

Table 10.5 Causes of lymph node enlargement

Infection
  Bacterial
    Acute, e.g. streptococcal, staphylococcal
    Chronic, e.g. tuberculosis
    Viral, e.g. infectious mononucleosis, cytomegalic inclusion disease, HIV
    Protozoan, e.g. toxoplasmosis

Neoplasm
  Lymphoma
  Leukaemia
  Carcinoma

Drugs
  Phenytoin

Others
  Autoimmune disease, e.g. systemic lupus erythematosus
  Sarcoidosis

and paradoxical excessive bleeding occur, and the patient may suffer from gout. A dusky cyanotic appearance is typical.

Other myeloproliferative disorders attract attention on account of various symptoms including pruritus, marrow failure and splenomegaly.

Myeloma

The clinical presentation is varied. The most common presenting symptom is bone pain, particularly in the lumbar and sacral regions. There may be bony tenderness and spontaneous fractures are common. In other cases the presenting feature may be anaemia, recurrent infections, chronic renal failure or a tendency to bleeding.

Leukaemia

Patients with acute leukaemia present with features of marrow failure; thus a tendency to bleeding, a propensity to infection and anaemia. Those with chronic lymphocytic leukaemia may notice enlargement of the lymph nodes.

Specific investigations

Investigations of the blood

Full blood count and blood film

In addition to the haemoglobin concentration and blood film, the initial blood examination should include total leucocyte and platelet counts and red cell absolute values. Electronic counters are now used extensively and these allow the rapid determination of the mean corpuscular volume (MCV), mean cell haemoglobin (MCH) and the mean cell haemoglobin concentration (MCHC).

The full blood count and blood film may show features of:

1 Anaemia.
  (a) Hypochromic microcytic blood film with thrombocytosis suggests iron deficiency.

Table 10.6 Causes of thrombocytopenia

Primary autoimmune
Drugs
Bone marrow disease
  Leukaemia
  Aplastic anaemia
  Infiltration—myelofibrosis, myeloma, lymphoma, secondary carcinoma
  Megaloblastic anaemia
Hypersplenism
Systemic lupus erythematosus
Infections
Disseminated intravascular coagulation

(b) Macrocytic megaloblastic picture with hypersegmentation of the neutrophils and thrombocytopenia typifies vitamin B_{12} or folic acid deficiency.

(c) Spherocytosis (very marked in hereditary spherocytosis) and reticulocytosis suggest a haemolytic anaemia. Fragmented red cells are found in microangiopathic haemolytic anaemia.

(d) Sickle-shaped cells occur in sickle cell anaemia.

(e) Target cells are aptly described and reflect thin cells which are found with severe iron deficiency, haemoglobinopathies and liver disease.

(f) Normochromic anaemia occurs in the presence of various inflammatory disorders representing infective, collagen or neoplastic disease. A marked degree of anisocytosis and poikilocytosis of the red cells and the presence of nucleated red cells is suggestive of marrow infiltration with malignant cells.

2   Red cell inclusions occur in various circumstances. Iron granules and nuclear remnants (Howell–Jolly bodies) are seen after splenectomy. Basophilic stippling suggests defective haemoglobin synthesis which occurs in lead poisoning and thalassaemia. Heinz bodies are precipitated haemoglobin (found after oxidative drug-induced haemolysis and in patients with glucose-6-phosphatase deficiency).

3   Depression of all three cell lines is indicative of marrow hypoplasia or hypersplenism. The leucocyte count tends to be low in SLE and in Felty's syndrome.

4   Thrombocytopenia; the causes of which are summarized in Table 10.6.

5   A high white cell count is commonly seen in chronic leukaemias, but the count is not necessarily high in acute leukaemia. Polymorph leucocytosis is typical of infection. It also occurs in some forms of vasculitis and after exposure to high dosages of corticosteroids.

6   Polycythaemia which may be secondary to chronic lung or cyanotic heart disease, or primary (polycythaemia rubra vera). In the latter case there is usually an increase in the platelet and white cell counts.

7   Evidence of alcohol abuse is frequently obtained. There is a macrocytosis and a depressed platelet count. Target cells may be evident in the presence of associated liver disease, when there may also be features of hyposplenism.

8   Malarial parasites can be a most important, if incidental, finding.

Erythrocyte sedimentation rate

The erythrocyte sedimentation rate (ESR) is an expression of the suspension stability of red cells in the blood. It is measured from the surface meniscus to the upper border of the red cell column after standing for 1 h. It depends on the specific gravity of the plasma and the propensity for red cells to clump (rouleaux formation) which is determined largely by fibrinogen.

The ESR is mainly used as a marker for the presence of organic disease, and occasionally to monitor disease activity during treatment. Elevated values are found in the elderly without obvious disease, and also in the presence of anaemia.

Particularly high values (>100 mm h^{-1}) occur in patients with vasculitis, e.g. cranial arteritis, and myeloma.

Viscosity is used as an alternative measurement in many centres.

Iron, transferrin and ferritin

The serum iron is low in patients with iron deficiency; it is also low in the presence of inflammatory disease. High levels may occur with other forms of hypochromic anaemia, such as thalassaemia, as well as in sideroblastic anaemia and states of iron overload.

Transferrin values are elevated with iron deficiency; they are normal in other forms of hypochromic or normochromic anaemia. Transferrin is also reduced by malnutrition.

Ferritin may more accurately reflect the iron status, and is particularly useful for the monitoring of patients who are undergoing regular venesection for the treatment of haemochromatosis.

Folate and vitamin B_{12}

These measurements are required in the presence of a macrocytic anaemia to distinguish deficiency from other causes such as ethanol abuse and marrow disorders.

Electrophoresis

Haemoglobin electrophoresis is required for the diagnosis of thalassaemia which may be suspected from a hypochromic blood film with an elevated serum iron in a patient with the appropriate family history. The haemoglobin electrophoresis shows increased amounts of HbA$_2$ and HbF.

Protein electrophoresis may disclose a monoclonal band in patients with myeloma.

Miscellaneous tests

Unconjugated bilirubin is increased during haemolysis when the blood haptoglobin is reduced. Under these circumstances measurement of the direct antiglobin test (Coombs test) and the red cell fragility should be considered. Increased fragility suggests spherocytosis; a positive Coombs test is indicative of autoimmune haemolytic anaemia.

Markers for SLE, the antinuclear factor and, if positive, DNA binding should be considered in patients with thrombocytopenia and lymphadenopathy. In the latter, the patient's serological markers for toxoplasma and Epstein–Barr infection (Paul–Bunnell test) may be needed. The possible need to screen for HIV infection and syphilis should not be overlooked.

The serum uric acid is increased in leukaemia and myeloproliferative disorders to the extent at which renal damage can occur if untreated. Serum urea may be high in myeloma and hypercalcaemia can contribute to the uraemia.

Bone marrow aspiration and trephine biopsy

Indications

Examination of the bone marrow is important in the diagnosis and management of a wide variety of diseases of the haemopoietic system. Indications include unexplained anaemia, leucopenia and thrombocytopenia and to assess the extent (or stage) of a variety of malignant conditions such as lymphoma. Aspiration of bone marrow is often sufficient to provide adequate diagnostic material; however, a trephine (or core) biopsy may be required if aspiration of marrow particles is unsuccessful, as may be the case in the presence of an infiltrated, fibrotic or hypercellular marrow. Trephine biopsy is also required as a staging procedure in lymphoma, for the definitive diagnosis of aplastic anaemia and in the investigation of a leucoerythroblastic anaemia when bone marrow metastases are being sought.

Sites

Accessible sites in adults include the sternal body, manubrium, anterior and posterior iliac spines, iliac crest and spinous processes. In children the preferred site is the posterior iliac spine, although in infants (less than 1 year old) a point on the anteromedial surface of the tibia 1–2 cm below the tibial tuberosity is perhaps easier. Trephine biopsy should only be carried out from the iliac crest or spines and *under no circumstances* be attempted from the sternum.

Procedure

The procedure should first be explained in full to the patient. In adults local anaesthesia is usually quite satisfactory but a brief general anaesthetic is usually preferred in children.

Microscopy of bone marrow smears stained with Romanosky dyes remains the most informative diagnostic procedure. A considerable amount of important additional information can be obtained from immunocytochemistry, chromosomal analysis, electron microscopy or cell culture. Various different fixatives or tissue culture media may therefore be required.

Use of radioisotopes

Radioactive vitamin B_{12}

The use of the simple and Dicopac-Schilling test to assess the absorption of vitamin B_{12} is described in Chapter 1.

Use of radioactive iron

The radioisotope of iron most commonly used is ^{59}Fe, which has a half-life of 45 days. The most useful diagnostic applications are the estimation of iron utilization from blood measurements and study of the site and magnitude of erythropoesis by surface counting.

Following the intravenous injection of a tracer dose of ^{59}Fe, given as ferric chloride solution, blood samples are collected at intervals for 2–3 weeks and the radioactivity of each blood sample is measured. The total red-cell volume must also be determined independently by the ^{51}Cr method. The total ^{59}Fe circulating in red cells as labelled haemoglobin can then be calculated and expressed as a percentage of the total injected radioactivity, thus giving a measure of the utilization of iron for haemoglobin. In the normal subject, the utilization reaches 70–80% after 10–14 days. In severe aplastic anaemia the maximum utilization may not exceed 10%.

When surface counting is being carried out, measurements are made over the liver, spleen and sacrum at intervals for 10–14 days after the injection of ^{59}Fe. In the normal subject the sacral activity rises rapidly over the first few hours as the iron enters the marrow, and then falls over the next 10 days as the red cells containing labelled haemoglobin enter the blood.

In aplastic anaemia there is poor uptake and release of radio-iron by the marrow, little uptake by the spleen and maximum uptake over the liver. In myelofibrosis, where there is extramedullary erythropoiesis, there may be very little change in the radioactivity counts over the sacrum, but the spleen may show an uptake and release of radioactivity indicating that it contains functioning erythropoietic tissue.

Use of radiochromium

^{51}Cr is used as a red-cell label in the measurement of total red-cell volume and of red-cell lifespan, in the detection of sites of red-cell destruction and in the quantitation of faecal blood loss.

In the measurement of total red-cell volume, a sample of venous blood is withdrawn and the red cells are incubated with a tracer dose of ^{51}Cr in the form of sodium chromate. The red cells are then washed, the radioactivity measured and a volume of the suspension of labelled red cells is re-injected intravenously. After allowing time for distribution and mixing throughout the circulation, further blood samples are taken after 10–20 min, for measurement of radioactivity. Knowing the radioactivity of the injected cells and of the subsequent samples, the degree of dilution of the labelled cells and hence the total circulating red-cell volume can be calculated. The normal total red-cell volume is 26–33 ml kg^{-1} in men and 22–29 ml kg^{-1} in women.

In the assessment of faecal blood loss, following the labelling and re-injection of a sample of the patient's red cells, the faeces are collected and the radio-activity measured. Knowing the radioactivity of the circulating blood, the volume of blood contained in each faecal collection can be calculated.

Red-cell lifespan can be studied by labelling and re-injecting a sample of the patient's own red cells and then taking blood samples at intervals until the radio-activity has fallen to less than half the initial level. In normal subjects the half-time for the disappearance of ^{51}Cr from the circulating blood is 26–30 days. In the absence of blood loss, a reduced ^{51}Cr half-time indicates a shortened red-cell lifespan due to a haemolytic process. In severe haemolytic anaemia, the ^{51}Cr half-time may be reduced to only a few days.

In the investigation of a patient with haemolytic anaemia, further information about the site of red-cell destruction can be obtained by surface counting over the heart, liver and spleen, following the injection of ^{51}Cr-labelled red cells. The observation of excessive accumulation of radioactivity occurring only in the spleen, indicating the primary site of red-cell destruction, may be of value in deciding whether to advise splenectomy in a case of haemolytic anaemia.

Tests for haemorrhagic disorders

Screening investigations

The initial investigation of any case of probable haemorrhagic disorder should include haemoglobin, blood film, leucocyte and platelet counts and bleeding time. Screening tests for coagulation factor deficiencies include the prothrombin time (PT) and activated partial thromboplastin time (APTT) (kaolin cephalin clotting time, KCCT).

Platelet count

Thrombocytopenia is defined as a platelet count below the normal range of $150 \times 10^9 \, l^{-1}$; bleeding is unlikely to be a problem with a platelet count above $100 \times 10^9 \, l^{-1}$. With counts in the region of $50 \times 10^9 \, l^{-1}$ spontaneous bleeding is uncommon but excessive bleeding may occur after trauma or surgery. Spontaneous bleeding may occur with counts of less than $30 \times 10^9 \, l^{-1}$ and may be severe when the count falls below $10 \times 10^9 \, l^{-1}$.

After confirming thrombocytopenia the cause must be established (see Table 10.6). In suspected autoimmune thrombocytopenia the detection of platelet antibodies is of value.

Bleeding time

The bleeding time is obtained by inflating a sphygmomanometer cuff on the upper arm to 40 mmHg. Using a spring lancet set at 3 mm, three skin punctures are made on the forearm. Blood from each puncture is removed with the edge of a filter paper every 15 s. The time to stop bleeding is normally 2.5–7 min. An alternative and more reliable method employs a template spring lancet which produces a standard incision 1 cm in length, with a normal value of up to 9 min.

The bleeding time is prolonged in thrombocytopenia, with qualitative platelet disorders, von Willebrand's disease, and in some cases of vascular purpura.

Tests of coagulation

1 PT reliably detects deficiencies of prothrombin and of factors V, VII and X.
The most common causes of prolongation are: (i) the effect of coumarin anticoagulant; (ii) hepatocellular disease with impaired synthesis of coagulation

factors; and (iii) deficiency of vitamin K due to malabsorption. Rarely, congenital deficiency of the above factors occurs; under these circumstances special assay of individual factors is needed.

2 Activated partial thromboplastin time (APTT): If PT is normal, a prolongation of this test is suggestive of either deficiency of factors VIII or IX, or the presence of an inhibitor, which may be the case in some patients with SLE.

3 Specific factor assays are occasionally required when individual deficiency is suspected; examples include the assay of factors VIII (haemophilia A) or factor IX (haemophilia B—Christmas disease).

Diagnostic approach

Suspected anaemia

Check the haemoglobin; if anaemic, check full blood count and film.

1 If hypochromic and microcytic, measure the iron and transferrin. If iron deficiency is confirmed consider: poor diet, menstrual losses, gastrointestinal cause (malabsorption and gastrointestinal bleeding, see p. 19).

If iron values are high consider: anaemia of inflammatory disorder (see below), thalassaemia and proceed to haemoglobin electrophoresis.

2 If normochromic and normocytic, consider: anaemia of chronic disorder (sometimes hypochromic and normocytic); measure the ESR or viscosity and screen for infective, neoplastic and collagen disease.

If haemolytic anaemia is suspected check bilirubin and haptoglobin; if in conjunction with the blood film the diagnosis is supported, then proceed to Coombs test, red-cell fragility.

3 If macrocytic, measure serum values for vitamin B_{12} and folic acid; if values are low, seek reasons, e.g. folate deficiency in diet, malabsorption of folate and vitamin B_{12} deficiency.

If values are normal seek other evidence of ethanol excess, e.g. thrombocytopenia and elevated serum enzymes, especially gamma-glutamyl transpeptidase. If negative consider examining the marrow.

Haemorrhagic disorder

1 Full blood count, especially platelet count.
2 Coagulation screen, including PT and KCCT.
3 Bleeding time.

Lymph node enlargement

1 Blood film; looking for evidence of infection, especially infectious mononucleosis, and leukaemia, especially chronic lymphatic.

2 Screen for infection, local or systemic, e.g. infectious mononucleosis with Paul–Bunnell test and possibly Epstein–Barr antibodies, toxoplasma and HIV antibodies.

3 Screen for sarcoidosis, e.g. Kveim test and for SLE by the ANF.

4 Excision biopsy and histological examination for malignancy and lymphoma.

Myeloproliferative disorders and leukaemia
1 Blood film.
2 Marrow examination.
3 Uric acid.
4 Suspected polycythaemia; red-cell mass and plasma volume.

Myeloma
1 Blood count.
2 Protein electrophoresis and 24-hour urine for Bence–Jones proteinuria.
3 Immunoglobulin values in serum.
4 Blood urea and creatinine.
5 Serum calcium.
6 Skeletal X-rays.
7 Marrow examination.

Chapter 11
Dermatology

Introduction

The investigation of any skin condition must begin with a careful history and full examination of the patient, not just a quick glance at the affected area. Failure to examine the feet or toe nails, the hair and mucous membranes may result in missed diagnoses. The duration and evolution of a rash, its colour, distribution and morphology often provides more information than most investigations. Conditions such as mild chronic plaque psoriasis, viral warts or scabies do not require investigation. In some inflammatory conditions, e.g. hand dermatitis, a trial of topical therapy together with general hand care instruction may be instituted initially and only if the condition fails to settle after a few weeks are investigations necessary (Fig. 11.1).

Observation of an atypical lesion over a period of time may allow diagnostic features to emerge or the rash to clear spontaneously. Other conditions demand immediate investigation, e.g. diagnostic biopsy in suspected malignant melanoma or culture of infected lesions, such as impetiginized dermatitis or 'eczema herpeticum'. Constant awareness of evidence for underlying systemic disease presenting with cutaneous signs is required. Foreign travel may result in the presentation of exotic diseases, such as leishmaniasis or tick typhus. Details of recent holidays, insect bites and contact with animals or household pets are important in assessing unusual-looking lesions.

General symptoms and signs

Symptoms

These may be either subjective and/or objective. Subjective sensations such as itch, pain, tingling or burning are common and can be severe. Diurnal variation can occur: itch is often worse at night, probably related to temperature. Tingling sensations precede the eruption in *Herpes simplex* or *H. zoster*. Symptoms are not always related to visible signs of disease—generalized pruritus may develop without a rash, although excoriations soon appear. Objective symptoms include visualization of a lesion which is otherwise asymptomatic, either by the patient, a relative or medical attendant. Lesions are sometimes felt initially, or come to light because they become irritated by clothing. There is increased awareness of skin lesions, especially pigmented ones, by the general public, prompted by publicity campaigns alerting people to early symptoms and signs of skin tumours. This is a common reason for presentation.

Signs

These are easily available and only require a good light and a careful observer. The range of pathology which the dermis and epidermis can express is limited

190

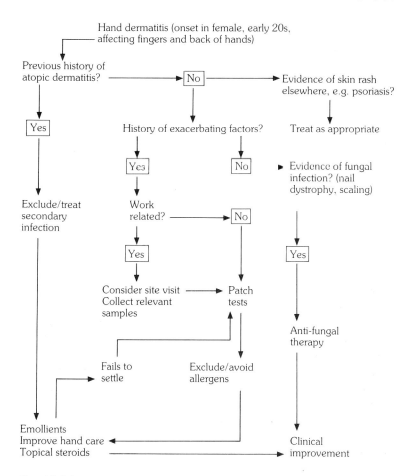

Fig. 11.1 Investigation of hand dermatitis.

but the clinical expression of those changes is surprisingly varied. Some lesions are diagnostic, such as the pearly nodule of a basal cell carcinoma or the scabetic burrow.

The morphology of lesions covers a range from macules (flat circumscribed lesions), papules and nodules, bullae (which may be tense or flaccid, on erythematous or normal skin, singly or in groups) and weals. Erythema and scaling are common features; secondary infection or excoriations modify appearances. Lichenification develops in excoriated skin in atopic dermatitis. Atropy, scarring, or diffuse thickening (as in morphoea), ulcers or changes in pigmentation may be present. Lesions may be distributed on various body sites, giving diagnostic information. For example, atopic dermatitis in older children is usually flexural whereas psoriasis often affects extensor surfaces. Involvement of hair and nails may be relevant. Widespread symmetrical eruptions may suggest a drug eruption. Contact dermatitis develops at the site of antigen exposure, e.g., the weight-bearing areas of the feet in shoe dermatitis, or sites in contact with jewellery or jeans studs in nickle dermatitis.

Specific investigations

Further investigations may be undertaken to clarify or assist with making a diagnosis, to identify any underlying associated disease or to document baseline indices before treatment. Most investigations are familiar, so only some of the more specialized procedures will be described.

1 Skin biopsy (light microscopy, immunofluorescence, special stains and electron microscopy).

2 Samples for microbiology (bacterial, mycological and virological).

3 Photography.

4 Patch testing, prick tests and other diagnostic skin tests.

5 Urinalysis.

6 Blood for haematological, biochemical and immunological testing.

7 Monitoring drug therapy.

8 Miscellaneous.

Skin biopsy

In most cases the histology of a biopsy specimen will establish, confirm or refute the clinical diagnosis. Planning the biopsy is important. Histology of an early lesion is more informative as secondary infection and excoriation may later mask underlying changes. Removal of a lesion requires attention to local anatomy and Langer's lines to reduce scarring. For a diagnostic biopsy, a representative lesion is selected, in a position which allows unimpeded healing and avoids areas of keloid predilection (presternum, shoulders and upper back). Punch biopsies are sufficient for some purposes, but an ellipse of skin, including normal and abnormal tissue, excised with a scalpel blade, is preferable. The size and depth of biopsy taken depends on the nature of the lesion and also on the investigations required. It may be necessary to divide tissue for different processing, e.g. formalin or glutaraldehyde fixation; fresh tissue is required for culture or processing for immunofluorescence studies. Completing the request form correctly helps the pathologist to make the diagnosis: the patient's age, the site and duration of the lesion, the nature of the rash, the working clinical diagnosis, the investigations required and details of previous biopsies are all important.

Immunofluorescence

Direct immunofluorescence detects the presence of antibody and complement components deposited in the skin. The biopsy should be taken from an early lesion, to include an intact blister if present, and tissue sent to the laboratory either fresh or snap-frozen. This test is a useful adjunct in the diagnosis of bullous disorders and connective tissue disorders.

Circulating antibodies to epidermal components present in the patient's serum can also be measured by indirect immunofluorescence, using a suitable substrate tissue.

Special stains

These are usually selected by the pathologist, based on information supplied on the request form. For example, fungal elements may be detected with a periodic acid–Schiff (PAS) stain; mast cells are more clearly visualized using toluidine blue stain and melanin deposits delineated with Fontana stain. Immunoperoxidase staining of monoclonal antibodies to cellular and tissue components is now widely used in research work and its use on diagnostic biopsies is likely to increase. Currently the technique is mainly used in the analysis of lymphocyte subsets in inflammatory and lymphomatous infiltrates.

Electron microscopy

This technique is essential in the diagnosis of the hereditary bullous diseases, e.g. epidermolysis bullosa, to establish the site of the abnormality in the dermo-epidermal junction. Fetoscopy and fetal skin biopsy enables prenatal diagnosis of severe forms of epidermolysis bullosa.

Electron microscopy can also be useful in identifying subcellular components, e.g. viruses or the Langerhan's cell granules present in the cellular infiltration of histiocytosis X (Letterer–Siwe disease).

Tissue culture

Fibroblasts cultured from biopsy tissue can be assessed for a number of functional abnormalities, e.g. chromosome repair mechanisms (abnormal in xeroderma pigmentosum) or defects in collagen synthesis (abnormal in Ehlers–Danlos syndrome).

Samples for microbiological investigations

Bacterial infection

Swabs from lesions are indicated if exudate or pus are present. A swab, moistened with sterile saline or water, can be used on a 'dry rash', e.g. atopic eczema. Crusts can be lifted off into transport medium; ulcer bases can be swabbed. Tissue from a biopsy may be required for diagnosis of, e.g. tuberculosis, leishmaniasis, leprosy, sporotrichosis or atypical mycobacterial infections. Interpretation of the results of skin swabs requires some knowledge of normal skin commensals and potential pathogens (Table 11.1). The quantity of the organism present may be important; for example, in atopic dermatitis Staphylococcus aureus is a common commensal, but exacerbations are often associated with increasing numbers of micro-organisms. Blood samples for culture, antistreptolysin-O (ASO) titres and fluorescent treponemal antibody absorption (FTA-ABS) tests may be required.

Viral infections

Swabs and blister fluid are appropriate for culture or electron microscopic diagnosis, where this is required. A biopsy can be helpful when the diagnosis is uncertain. Paired samples (acute and convalescent) of venous blood for viral titres may be useful. Blood samples for serology are also indicated if hepatitis B or HIV infections are suspected.

Fungal infections

Fungal elements are found in epidermal keratin. Thus, nail clippings, plucked hairs and scrapings from the skin surface are appropriate. Scrapings can be

Table 11.1 Normal skin commensals

Corynebacteria
  'Diphtheroids—gram-positive rods, aerobic or anaerobic,
  e.g. *Corynebacterium acnes*.

Micrococcaceae
  Gram-positive cocci*, e.g. *Staphylococcus albus*.

Streptococci
  Gram-positive cocci, mainly α and γ haemolytic

Gram-negative bacilli
  E.g. *Proteus*, present in 5–15% normals (nose and toe webs)

Pityrosporum ovale
  Yeast; in association with sebaceous glands, on the scalp

Candida spp.
  Including *C. albicans*

Demodex folliculorum
  Mite associated with hair follicles and sebaceous glands, especially on the face

* *Staphylococcus aureus* is present in 5–15% normals (nose, perineum, toe webs).

obtained using a scalpel blade held at 45° to the skin surface and literally scraping the skin surface firmly. Scrapings should be collected into a piece of folded paper or onto microscope slides which can be taped together for transport to the laboratory, where direct microscopy is performed and cultures are set up. Direct microscopy may be useful in the clinic: scrapings should be placed on a slide with a few drops of 10% potassium hydroxide solution and warmed slightly before viewing, looking for hyphae and spores amongst the keratinocytes.

Yeast infections

Candida albicans can be detected by taking swabs for culture.

Wood's lamp (an ultraviolet light source from which visible light has been excluded by a nickel oxide filter) can be used to detect some fungal infections; brilliant green fluorescence is induced in scalp infections due to *Microsporum canis* and *M. audouinii* and a paler green fluorescence with *Trichophyton schoenleinii*. Infections such as erythrasma produce a coral-pink fluorescence.

Infestations

Nits and adult forms of lice are generally visible to the naked eye. The diagnosis of scabies is essentially clinical, but may be confirmed by finding an acaris and viewing it under the microscope.

Where more specialized data is required, such as typing of human papilloma viruses or herpes viruses, or phage typing, e.g. *Staphylococcus aureus*, liaison with the laboratory is advised. Investigations for immune deficiency or diabetes mellitus should be carried out in patients with persistent or unusual skin infections, or other cutaneous manifestations in, e.g. homosexuals or drug addicts.

Photography

It is often important to document carefully the nature and extent of a rash or lesions. The evolution of lesions or changes as a result of therapy can be followed with serial photographs.

Patch testing

This investigation is undertaken when contact dermatitis resulting from an environmental (external) allergen is suspected. The object of patch testing is to reproduce, in a controlled manner, a delayed hypersensitivity response to an allergen applied to the surface of the skin. The suspect allergen is applied under special occlusive chambers and left in place for at least 48 h. A positive test will show erythema and induration, and possibly blistering at the point of contact with the allergen within 48–72 h. If such a reaction is biopsied, the characteristic perivascular lymphohistiocytic inflammatory infiltrate of a delayed hypersensitivity response can be observed.

There is a vast range of potential allergens known to cause contact dermatitis: this investigation must be used with logic and common sense, based on the clinical history, the presence of an appropriate rash and knowledge of relevant potential sensitizers. The history should include details of work and home factors thought to aggravate the rash; the site of the rash may provide clues. In practice, standard batteries of potentially sensitizing compounds are available. The standard European battery forms the basis of most patch-test routines and contains about 30 of the common sensitizers (Table 11.2).

Specialized batteries are available for certain 'at risk' groups, e.g. hairdressers. More complex problems may require a visit to the place of work to obtain samples of work materials for testing. Work-related disease raises potential medico-legal problems and care should be taken in the interpretation of results. Some substances provoke an irritant reaction on the skin, which is not easily distinguished from an allergic reaction. Test substances should be applied in the optimum concentration to avoid irritation occurring. A positive reaction which does not in any way relate to the patient's problem should be viewed with caution. Since the

Table 11.2 Common causes of contact dermatitis

Compound	Present in
Nickel sulphate	Coins, metal plated objects, e.g. jewellery
Paraphenylene diamine (PPD)	Hair and textile dyes
Formaldehyde Chlorocresol Ethylene diamine Parabens Wool alcohols (lanolin)	Preservatives, stabilizers or bases for ointments or creams
Chinoform Neomycin	Topical antiseptics and antibiotics
Thiuram-mix Mercapto-mix Carba-mix PPD-mix	Rubber additives

chemicals are potential sensitizers, care should be taken by the handler to avoid unnecessary contact at the time of application. Photo-patch testing is an additional technique which can be used to diagnose photo-allergic and photo-toxic disorders. These investigations are carried out in specialist centres, using a combination of standard patch testing and exposure to varying wavelengths of ultraviolet light.

IgE levels and radio-allergosorbent tests

In atopic dermatitis, the level of IgE is often, but not always, raised. It is usually highest in patients with associated asthma. IgE levels do not reflect the severity of the rash nor its response to treatment. Radio-allergosorbent tests (RAST) record levels of specific IgE and may indicate potential sensitizers such as house-dust mites, animal danders or certain foods; often these will have been suggested by the history. In practice, these results may not be of any value in the management of the dermatitis and it is important to avoid domestic or dietary manoeuvres which disrupt the patient's life unnecessarily.

Prick tests and other diagnostic skin tests

Prick skin tests, using standard batteries of allergen extracts, are available. A drop of the solution is placed on the skin, which is then gently scratched with a needle. Positive results show a weal and flare response within 20 min. Although these tests may be useful in hay fever or asthma, they are not generally useful in atopic dermatitis; frequent false positive tests produce an apparently wide range of potential allergens—exclusion of these substances seldom produces clinical improvement.

Other diagnostic skin tests include the Mantoux and Kveim tests, trichophytin and lepromin tests. The basis of these tests is the introduction of specific antigen into the dermis. Clinical reactions are measured at pre-determined times (e.g. 48 or 72 h for the Mantoux and trichophytin tests). The Kveim test site is biopsied to confirm the presence of an appropriate granulomatous inflammatory response after a period of 6 weeks. The lepromin test has an early (Fernandez–48 h) and a late (Mitsuda–4 weeks) component. The test material must be injected into the dermis, not subcutaneously. Careful measurement of the erythema and induration should be done in the long axis of the forearm and at right angles, with results expressed as the mean of the two diameters. Natural skin markings, e.g. melanonaevi, should be used where possible when documenting the site of a Kveim test for future biopsy.

Urinalysis

Screening patients for diabetes mellitus is important since previously undiagnosed cases may present to the dermatologist. Many skin conditions, such as generalized pruritus, recurrent bacterial or yeast infections, leg ulcers (vascular or neurotrophic) and eruptive xanthomata are common in diabetics. Granuloma annulare and necrobiosis lipoidica may be associated with a family history of diabetes. Haematuria and/or proteinuria may be evidence of renal involvement in patients with systemic disease, e.g. SLE, scleroderma, sarcoidosis. It is also found in drug eruptions, Henoch–Schönlein purpura and should be looked for in patients with streptococcal skin infection. Unexplained positive findings should be followed by repeat testing and a mid-stream specimen of urine (MSU).

Blood tests for haematological, biochemical and immunological indices

This section is intended to emphasize the close relationship between dermatological and systemic disease. Examples of both haematological and biochemical abnormalities associated with skin disorders, and cutaneous signs of haematological and biochemical disorders are included.

Haematological abnormalities

Severe cutaneous infections will be accompanied by a raised erythrocyte sedimentation rate (ESR) and increased white cell count (polymorphonuclear leucocytes or lymphocytes) depending on the nature of the infection. Eosinophilia occurs in both infective and allergic disorders, e.g. parasitic infections and drug eruptions. Polycythaemia rubra vera may present with generalized pruritus. In cold-related disorders cryoglobulins should be looked for; this requires a fresh sample, taken to the laboratory while still warm. In patients with thrombotic episodes and livedo reticularis prolongation of the kaolin cephalin clotting test (KCCT) suggests the presence of a 'lupus anticoagulant' antibody. This is confirmed by the detection of anticardiolipin antibodies. Some dermatological disorders and cutaneous signs which may be associated with haematological abnormalities are shown in Table 11.3.

Table 11.3 Signs suggesting haematological abnormalities

Signs	Possible laboratory findings
Koilonychia, pallor, angular stomatitis, diffuse hair loss	Iron deficiency anaemia
Familial haemorrhagic telangiectasia, blue rubber bleb naevus syndrome, pseudoxanthoma elasticum, Ehlers–Danlos syndrome, Peutz–Jeghers syndrome	Possible causes of gastrointestinal blood loss and consequent anaemia
Vitiligo	Association with pernicious anaemia
Dermatitis herpetiformis with gluten enteropathy	Folate deficiency
Purpuric lesions Generalized lesions (petechiae, ecchymoses, mucous membrane bleeding)	Thrombocytopenia
Henloch–Schönlein purpura (palpable): extensor aspect legs, arms, buttocks	Vasculitis
Senile purpura Scurvy	Deficient collagen support, vessel fragility
Skin fragility with blisters on light-exposed areas	Porphyria
Cryoglobulinaemia, multiple myeloma	Dysproteinaemias
Bruising *or* bleeding diathesis	Coagulation factor deficiency e.g. haemophilia A *or* B
Bruising *and* unexplained injuries	Non-accidental injury: (normal haematology)

Biochemical abnormalities

Urea, electrolytes and creatinine

Mild derangement of renal function is not uncommon in patients with chronic venous insufficiency and varicose ulcers on diuretic therapy. Many of these patients are also on digoxin. Erythroderma (of various causes, e.g. psoriasis, dermatitis, drug eruptions) may be associated with severe fluid and electrolyte disturbances. As mentioned earlier, renal involvement may develop in patients with, for example, SLE. These tests are also important when monitoring drug therapy (see Table 11.4).

Table 11.4 Monitoring drug therapy

Drug	Investigation	Possible complications
Methotrexate*	Full blood count and film	Macrocytic (folate deficiency) anaemia Hypoplastic *or* aplastic anaemia Agranulocytosis, thrombocytopenia
	Urea and electrolytes, creatinine	Toxicity increased if renal function impaired
	Liver function tests Liver biopsy (after each 2 g *or* before if serum biochemistry is abnormal	Can cause hepatic fibrosis and possibly cirrhosis
Azathioprine	Full blood count and film Liver function tests	Agranulocytosis Aplastic anaemia Drug-induced hepatitis
Retinoid drugs† (etretinate; isoretinoin)	Fasting lipids Liver function tests	Elevations of triglyceride *and/or* cholesterol Hepatotoxic
Corticosteroids‡ (prednisolone)	Urea, electrolytes Blood sugar	Hypertension Obesity Diabetes mellitus Peptic ulceration
Oxytetracycline	Urea, electrolytes, creatinine	Contra-indicated in renal and hepatic failure, pregnancy, young children
8-Methoxypsoralens (for PUVA therapy)	Urea, electrolytes, creatinine Liver function tests Antinuclear antibody Ophthalmological assessment	Contra-indicated in renal and hepatic failure Contra-indicated in SLE or pregnancy
Dapsone§	Full blood count and film	Haemolytic anaemia Aplastic anaemia Agranulocytosis

* (a) Interactions with many non-steroidal anti-inflammatory drugs potentiate toxicity.
   (b) Once weekly oral dose minimizes side-effects.
† Consider pregnancy test pre-treatment; teratogenic.
‡ Measure blood pressure and weight pre-treatment.
§ Glucose-6-phosphate dehydrogenase status should be considered.

Liver function tests

The combination of chronic skin disorders and alcoholism is common, especially in patients with psoriasis. Most systemic drugs used to treat psoriasis are metabolized in the liver or cause hepatic damage and are thus contra-indicated if liver damage is already present due to alcohol. Erythema nodosum or urticaria and arthralgia may occur during the prodromal phase of viral hepatitis (usually type B). Patients with recent tattoos may be at risk of developing this infection. The stigmata of chronic liver disease, gynaecomastia, spider naevi and palmar erythema, are well recognized. Primary biliary cirrhosis may present with generalized pruritus and widely excoriated skin, or with xanthomas. Investigation of abnormal pigmentation will include consideration of the slate-grey pigmentation of haemochromatosis.

Cholesterol and triglyceride levels

In isolation, xanthelasma and juvenile xanthogranulomata are not usually associated with lipid abnormalities. Other xanthomata are more commonly associated with abnormal blood lipids. The demonstration of raised cholesterol or triglycerides in a fasting blood sample should be followed by exclusion of secondary causes of hyperlipidaemia (hypothyroidism, diabetes mellitus, obstructive liver disease, nephrotic syndrome or dysproteinaemias) and classification of the abnormality if primary.

Muscle enzyme analysis

The characteristic features of dermatomyositis (poikilodermatous rash with heliotrope discoloration around the eyes, Gottron's papules on the fingers and proximal muscle weakness) are well recognized. Elevations of creatine kinase may be transient if the myositis is not prominent. If the diagnosis is established, a search for underlying malignant disease is required in older patients.

Complement components

Low complement components, especially C_3 may be seen in patients with active SLE. Recurrent angioedema, either familial or acquired (usually in association with lymphoid or myeloid disease) may be due to deficiency of C_1 esterase inhibitor. This deficiency is variable in the acquired group and associated with low C_1 levels too.

Thyroid function tests

Cutaneous manifestations occur in both hyperthyroidism (diffuse hair loss, pruritus, acropachy and pre-tibial myxoedema) and hypothyroidism (dry skin, oedema of the face, hands and feet, loss of body hair and coarse scalp hair). Thyroid function tests (T4, T3 and TSH) may be indicated.

Sex hormone assay

Hirsutism, as distinct from hypertrichosis, should be initially investigated with measurement of serum testosterone and androstenedione. Assessment of ovarian function, including ovarian ultrasound and assessment of cyclic patterns of luteinizing hormone (LH) and follicle-stimulating hormone (FSH) levels to

Table 11.5 Pattern of porphyrin abnormalities in some porphyrias (acute phase)

Sample	Porphyrin metabolite	Type of porphyria		
		EPP	PCT	VP
Red blood cells	Protoporphyrin	↑	N	N
Urine	Δ-amino-laevulinic acid	N	N	↑
	Porphobilinogen	N	N	↑
	Uroporphyrin	N	↑	↑
	Coproporphyrin	N	↑	↑
Faeces	Coproporphyrin	N	N	↑
	Protoporphyrin	↑	N	↑

Abbreviations: EPP = erythropoietic protoporphyria; PCT = porphyria cutanea tarda; VP = variegate porphyria; N = normal *or* absent; ↑ = raised.

detect the polycystic ovary syndrome, require more specialized facilities. Other causes of hirsutism include ovarian or adrenal tumours and occasionally drug therapy, e.g. minoxidil, diazoxide. Patients presenting with striae may need to have Cushing's disease excluded.

Porphyrin metabolites

The diagnosis and classification of the porphyrias involves measuring levels of the various porphyrin metabolites in red blood cells, faeces and urine. Fresh samples are needed for the analysis and liaison with the laboratory is desirable. The common abnormalities detected are shown in Table 11.5.

Immunological abnormalities

Organ specific autoantibodies

Vitiligo may be associated with other autoimmune disorders and the relevant autoantibodies should be looked for in the peripheral blood. In bullous pemphigoid, circulating anti-basement antibodies may be present while in pemphigus, anti-intercellular substance antibodies can be measured, the titre paralleling clinical progress.

Non-organ specific antibodies

These are usually found in the context of connective tissue diseases. The screening test for SLE is the antinuclear antibody. Other serological markers, such as DNA (native or single-stranded), Ro or La antibodies may be present. Patients with cutaneous lupus erythematosus (LE), sometimes called discoid LE, do not generally have positive serology. The localized cutaneous form of scleroderma (morphoea) is seldom associated with positive serology. Antinuclear antibodies may be found in up to 90% of patients with progressive systemic sclerosis; antinucleolar antibody is present in about 50% of cases, as are anticentromere antibodies with the calcinosis, Raynaud's phenomenon, sclerodactyly, telangiectasis (CRST) syndrome. In rheumatoid arthritis, extra-articular manifestations, such as nodules or vasculitic lesions, are commonly associated with seropositivity, the severity of lesions reflecting the antibody titre. The detection of circulating immune complexes may aid the diagnosis of some allergic or vasculitic disorders.

Monitoring drug therapy

Investigations should be directed towards detecting likely complications at appropriate intervals during therapy. Some of the systemic agents used by dermatologists are listed in Table 11.4, together with their more common side-effects and appropriate investigations.

Miscellaneous investigations

Simple tests of skin function, such as sweat or sebum production, and skin blood flow, can be performed and a variety of techniques is available to assess epidermal kinetics.

The diagnosis of systemic diseases presenting with cutaneous lesions may require more extensive investigation than has been outlined in this chapter.

Diagnostic approach

This section tabulates the use of diagnostic techniques in selected dermatological conditions. The nature of dermatology is such that investigation is frequently unnecessary, e.g. the patient with mild classical psoriasis or with acquired scabies. Conversely, the elucidation of the cause of dermatitis can be tedious. Such a problem is illustrated in Fig. 11.1.

Hand dermatitis

Consider:

1 *Screen for infections*, e.g. bacterial and fungal.
2 *Patch tests* for allergens.

Urticaria

Consider:

1 *Screen for infections*, e.g. full blood count, stools for ova and parasites, urine for analysis and culture, vaginal inspection for *Candida*, X-ray of chest and sinuses.
2 *Cold urticaria*—cryoglobulins and ice-cube provocation test.
3 *Solar urticaria*—photo-testing with solar simulator.
4 *Cholinergic urticaria*—mecholyl skin test.
5 *Foods*—elimination and re-addition diets. Immediate scratch and intradermal skin tests.
6 *RAST*.

Pruritus of unknown cause

Consider:

1 *Chronic cholestasis*—liver function tests.
2 *Anaemia*—blood count, iron and transferrin.
3 *Diabetes*—blood glucose.
4 *Worm infestation*—stools for ova and parasites.
5 *Lymphoma*—skin biopsy and chest X-ray.

Dermatitis herpetiformis
Consider:
1 *Biopsy* for histology and immunofluoresence.
2 *Screen for malabsorption*, e.g. blood count and, if anaemic, folate and vitamin B_{12}.
3 *Jejunal biopsy.*

Erythema multiforme
Consider
1 *Infective agents*, e.g. mycoplasma or viral serology.
2 *Drugs*—history.
3 *Collagen vascular disease*—antinuclear factors (ANF), ESR, etc.
4 *Malignant disease*—chest X-ray, latex fixation test (LFT), full blood count (FBC).

Erythema nodosum
Consider:
1 *Infections*—throat swab and antistreptolysin-O titre.
2 *Sarcoidosis*—chest X-ray, Kveim test.
3 *Tuberculosis*—chest X-ray.
4 *Sputum for acid fast bacilli*—renal or gastrointestinal investigations, if indicated.
5 *Inflammatory bowel disease*—sigmoidoscopy, barium examinations, if indicated.

Cutaneous sarcoid
1 *Biopsy* for histology.
2 *Chest X-ray and pulmonary function tests.*
3 *Blood urea and calcium.*

Chapter 12
Nutrition

Introduction

Nutrition is relevant in every branch of medical practice, undernutrition, overnutrition and inappropriate nutrition are all major factors in the pathogenesis of disease.

Many studies have shown that undernutrition is common in both medical and surgical hospital practice. Frequently, the nutritional status deteriorates during the course of the hospital stay. This is particularly true of general surgery, gastroenterology and oncology. Malnutrition in this form is a serious problem which greatly enhances morbidity and mortality. It is associated with increased susceptibility to infection, delayed wound healing and an apathetic, withdrawn patient who is unable to co-operate satisfactorily with treatment and who is ultimately regarded as depressed.

Obesity is also a cause of increased morbidity. These patients are prone to an increased incidence of various diseases (Table 12.1).

Recently, interest has focused on the role that nutrition may play in the pathogenesis of many degenerative diseases. Obvious examples include: the consumption of saturated fats and their association with vascular disease; intake of salt and alcohol linked to hypertension; and refined diets in association with diverticular disease.

General symptoms

Obesity

Many authorities define overweight and obesity as weights which are respectively 10% and 20% above the upper limits of an accepted weight range (Table 12.2). Such definitions take no account of the relative contributions of muscle mass and adipose tissue. Inspection will reveal the truth to most observers!

Malnutrition

Protein–energy malnutrition

Patients who restrict their diet, either to avoid distressing intestinal symptoms in the presence of abdominal disease or on account of anorexia nervosa, become

Table 12.1 Diseases associated with obesity

Diabetes mellitus	Gout
Hypertension	Pulmonary disease
Coronary heart disease	Hernias
Cholelithiasis	Varicose veins
Osteoarthrosis	Intertrigo

Table 12.2 1983 Metropolitan height and weight tables for men and women on metric basis, according to frame, ages 25–59.

Height (in shoes)† (cm)	Men (weight in kg [in indoor clothing])*			
	Small frame	Medium frame	Midpoint	Large frame
158	58.3–61.0	59.6–64.2	61.9	62.8–68.3
159	58.6–61.3	59.9–64.5	62.2	63.1–68.8
160	59.0–61.7	60.3–64.9	62.6	63.5–69.4
161	59.3–62.0	60.6–65.2	62.9	63.8–69.9
162	59.7–62.4	61.0–65.6	63.3	64.2–70.5
163	60.0–62.7	61.3–66.0	63.7	64.5–71.1
164	60.4–63.1	61.7–66.5	64.1	64.9–71.8
165	60.8–63.5	62.1–67.0	64.6	65.3–72.5
166	61.1–63.8	62.4–67.6	65.0	65.6–73.2
167	61.5–64.2	62.8–68.2	65.5	66.0–74.0
168	61.8–64.6	63.2–68.7	66.0	66.4–74.7
169	62.2–65.2	63.8–69.3	66.6	67.0–75.4
170	62.5–65.7	64.3–69.8	67.1	67.5–76.1
171	62.9–66.2	64.8–70.3	67.6	68.0–76.8
172	63.2–66.7	65.4–70.8	68.1	68.5–77.5
173	63.6–67.3	65.9–71.4	68.7	69.1–78.2
174	63.9–67.8	66.4–71.9	69.2	69.6–78.9
175	64.3–68.3	66.9–72.4	69.7	70.1–79.6
176	64.7–68.9	67.5–73.0	70.3	70.7–80.3
177	65.0–69.5	68.1–73.5	70.8	71.3–81.0
178	65.4–70.0	68.6–74.0	71.3	71.8–81.8
179	65.7–70.5	69.2–74.6	71.9	72.3–82.5
180	66.1–71.0	69.7–75.1	72.4	72.8–83.3
181	66.6–71.6	70.2–75.8	73.0	73.4–84.0
182	67.1–72.1	70.7–76.5	73.6	73.9–84.7
183	67.7–72.7	71.3–77.2	74.3	74.5–85.4
184	68.2–73.4	71.8–77.9	74.9	75.2–86.1
185	68.7–74.1	72.4–78.6	75.5	75.9–86.8
186	69.2–74.8	73.0–79.3	76.2	76.6–87.6
187	69.8–75.5	73.7–80.0	76.9	77.3–88.5
188	70.3–76.2	74.4–80.7	77.6	78.0–89.4
189	70.9–76.9	74.9–81.5	78.2	78.7–90.3
190	71.4–77.6	75.4–82.2	78.8	79.4–91.2
191	72.1–78.4	76.1–83.0	79.6	80.3–92.1
192	72.8–79.1	76.8–83.9	80.4	81.2–93.0
193	73.5–79.8	77.6–84.8	81.2	82.1–93.9

* Indoor clothing weighing 2.3 kg for men and 1.4 kg for women.
† Shoes with 2.5 cm heels. Reproduced from *Statistical Bulletin* (1983). Metropolitan Life Insurance Company, New York.

Table 12.2 (cont.)

| Height (in shoes)† (cm) | Women (weight in kg [in indoor clothing])* | | | |
	Small frame	Medium frame	Midpoint	Large frame
148	46.4–50.6	49.6–55.1	52.4	53.7–59.8
149	46.6–51.0	50.0–55.5	52.3	54.1–60.3
150	46.7–51.3	50.3–55.9	53.1	54.4–60.9
151	46.9–51.7	50.7–56.4	53.6	54.8–61.4
152	47.1–52.1	51.1–57.0	54.1	55.2–61.9
153	47.4–52.5	51.5–57.5	54.5	55.6–62.4
154	47.8–53.0	51.9–58.0	55.0	56.2–63.0
155	48.1–53.6	52.2–58.6	55.4	56.8–63.6
156	48.5–54.1	52.7–59.1	55.9	57.3–64.1
157	48.8–54.6	53.2–59.6	56.4	57.8–64.6
158	49.3–55.2	53.8–60.2	57.0	58.4–65.3
159	49.8–55.7	54.3–60.7	57.5	58.9–66.0
160	50.3–56.2	54.9–61.2	58.1	59.4–66.7
161	50.8–56.7	55.4–61.7	58.6	59.9–67.4
162	51.4–57.3	55.9–62.3	59.1	60.5–68.1
163	51.9–57.8	56.4–62.8	59.6	61.0–68.8
164	52.5–58.4	57.0–63.4	60.2	61.5–69.5
165	53.0–58.9	57.5–63.9	60.7	62.0–70.2
166	53.6–59.5	58.1–64.5	61.3	62.6–70.9
167	54.1–60.0	58.7–65.0	61.9	63.2–71.7
168	54.6–60.5	59.2–65.5	62.4	63.7–72.4
169	55.2–61.1	59.7–66.1	62.9	64.3–73.1
170	55.7–61.6	60.2–66.6	63.4	64.8–73.8
171	56.2–62.1	60.7–67.1	63.9	65.3–74.5
172	56.8–62.6	61.3–67.6	64.5	65.8–75.2
173	57.3–63.2	61.8–68.2	65.0	66.4–75.9
174	57.8–63.7	62.3–68.7	65.5	66.9–76.4
175	58.3–64.2	62.8–69.2	66.0	67.4–76.9
176	58.9–64.8	63.4–69.8	66.6	68.0–77.5
177	59.5–65.4	64.0–70.4	67.2	68.5–78.1
178	60.0–65.9	64.5–70.9	67.7	69.0–78.6
179	60.5–66.4	65.1–71.4	68.3	69.6–79.1
180	61.0–66.9	65.6–71.9	68.8	70.1–79.6
181	61.6–67.5	66.1–72.5	69.3	70.7–80.2
182	62.1–68.0	66.6–73.0	69.8	71.2–80.7
183	62.6–68.5	67.1–73.5	70.3	71.7–81.2

wasted with loss of adipose tissue and muscle bulk, but the serum albumin concentration is maintained. Conversely, patients who are stressed with burns or sepsis appear less wasted but they suffer a rapid loss of their muscle bulk and develop hypo-albuminaemia. Such muscle wasting is seen most readily around the shoulder girdle. Too often it is overlooked, particularly in the obese subject, until malnutrition has reached an advanced stage.

Micronutrient deficiency

Vitamins

Vitamin A deficiency has a major impact on the eye. Night blindness may be followed by xerophthalmia and corneal damage. The role of this vitamin in the maintenance of the integrity of the epithelium is important in relation to protection against infection.

Thiamin deficiency may develop in hospital practice because body stores only amount to 1 month's provision. Deficiency is characterized by neurological features such as the Wernicke–Korsakoff syndrome or polyneuropathy, or biventricular cardiac failure.

Niacin depletion is characterized by diarrhoea, dermatitis and dementia. Deficiency of vitamin B_{12} affects the marrow leading to a megaloblastic anaemia (likewise folic acid), and affects the neurological system with peripheral neuropathy or subacute combined degeneration of the cord.

Vitamin C deficiency has long been associated with scurvy, and deficiency of vitamin D with rickets and osteomalacia.

Trace elements

Zinc deficiency may readily occur because of limited body stores. It leads to dermatitis and diarrhoea and, in children, dwarfism and hypogonadism.

Recent interest has focused on selenium deficiency, which can cause a myopathy, including cardiomyopathy.

Depletion of copper has been associated with leucopenia and neutropenia. In children, bone changes and growth impairment also occur, with sparse brittle hair, arterial and cerebral degeneration.

In all malnourished patients in this country the clinical features of malnutrition may be variably masked by those of the underlying disease which frequently distracts attention from the nutritional problem. When malnutrition is found in underdeveloped countries it is usually accompanied and aggravated by secondary infection.

Specific investigations

Dietary assessment

Dietary assessment is used for two reasons: (i) to establish the adequacy of the diet; and (ii) to gain insight into the patient's eating practice so that therapeutic diets may be devised to suit his or her convenience.

There are three methods which are commonly used.

Dietary recall

The patient is asked to remember the food that has been eaten over the previous day or longer. This is an inaccurate method because of the fallibility of the patient's memory and the self-delusion of the obese!

Preferred foods

Patients are asked to list their likes and dislikes in terms of food items and meals. This gives some insights into the nature of the diet, more particularly in terms of foods which may not be considered appropriate.

Food weighing

The only accurate method of dietary assessment involves itemizing and weighing each food portion as it is consumed—a tedious task that requires an obsessional and conscientious patient!

Nutritional requirements

Accepted nutritional requirements may be obtained from standard nutritional texts. However, the needs of the ill and stressed patient have been poorly defined and are likely to differ from those that currently apply to the healthy subject. Accurate measurement of the energy needs of individual patients can be made by recording oxygen consumption and carbon dioxide production. This is a research technique which is not available in clinical practice. For routine management, calculations based on the Harris–Benedict formula, as shown below, serve as a rough guide.

To estimate energy requirements:

1 Calculate basal energy expenditure (BEE) using Harris–Benedict formula,

Male BEE $= 66.47 + 13.75(W) + 5.0(H) - 6.75(A)$
Female BEE $= 65.51 + 9.56(W) + 1.85(H) - 4.68(A)$

where W = weight in kg, H = height in cm, and A = age in years.

2 Adjust for activity and injury factors.

Activity factor:	Bed rest	1.2
	Out of bed	1.3
Injury factor:	Minor surgery	1.2
	Skeletal trauma	1.35
	Major sepsis	1.6
	Burns	2.0

3 Adjust for nutritional goal.

Stressed patient—maintain weight.

Nutritional repletion—add up to 4200 kJ per day.

Knowledge about protein, as well as energy, requirements is important during the treatment of ill, undernourished patients. Nitrogen balance is usually measured, principally from urea excretion, as shown below.

Nitrogen loss (g) = mmol urinary urea per 24 h $\times$ 0.028 + 2
+ change in blood urea per 24 h (mmol) $\times$ 0.028 $\times$ 0.6
$\times$ W + urinary protein loss (g) − 6.25.

Anthropometric measurements

Weight and height

Patients should be weighed without clothing at the same time each day. Rapid fluctuations in weight reflect changes in fluid balance rather than nutritional status.

Changes in growth velocity indicate changes in nutritional state or disease activity. Accurate measurements of height are essential in paediatric practice.

Body mass index

This is a simple index derived statistically from population data on weights and heights. It is measured by the formula:

$$\frac{\text{weight (kg)}}{[\text{height (m)}]^2}$$

This index is most commonly used as a marker of obesity. Normal values are below 25.

Skin fold thickness

This is used as a simple measure of body fat. Because of racial differences in fat distribution, the sum of skin-fold thickness measured at four sites is used as an index of adiposity. These sites are: triceps, biceps, subscapular and supra-iliac crest. Normal values range from 40–80 mm.

When skin-fold thickness is being used to identify undernutrition and monitor response to treatment, the triceps measurement alone is sufficient (Table 12.3).

Mid-arm muscle circumference

This measurement is used as a simple index of body muscle. It is influenced by oedema and variations in technique. It is derived from the formula:

Muscle circumference = arm circumference (cm)
              – triceps skin-fold thickness (mm).

Values of arm muscle circumference are given in Table 12.3.

Table 12.3 Adult standards for anthropometric measurements

	Triceps skin fold thickness (mm)		
	Standard	80% of standard	60% of standard
Male	12.5	10.0	7.7
Female	16.5	13.2	9.9

	Arm muscle circumference (cm)		
	Standard	80% of standard	60% of standard
Male	25.3	20.2	15.2
Female	23.2	18.6	13.9

Reproduced from Pennington C.R. (1988) *Therapeutic Nutrition*. Chapman & Hall Ltd, London.

Dynamometry

Muscle function is a more sensitive index of impaired nutrition than muscle size; thus the measurement of grip strength using a dynamometer is used to assess malnutrition. However, results are dependent on the patient's willingness to co-operate.

Laboratory measurement

Biochemistry

Proteins

Serum albumin and transferrin provide evidence of visceral protein status. The half-life of albumin is 16–18 days and that for transferrin 6–8 days. Whereas increasing values, first for transferrin and followed by albumin, may indicate improving nutritional status in the stable patient, fluid shifts and loss of proteins from the vascular space make interpretation difficult.

Electrolytes

Significant disturbance of water and electrolyte balance is a common feature in severe malnutrition, particularly in patients who have trauma, sepsis or multisystem disease. Abnormalities of sodium, potassium, magnesium and pH may require correction.

Minerals and trace elements

Serum values of calcium, magnesium, zinc and iron are routinely available. However, the measurement of trace elements such as selenium and chromium is more difficult and requires a supra-regional service.

Vitamins

Measurement of vitamins is also less widely available. Some of the methods employed are shown in Table 12.4

Table 12.4 Some laboratory methods used for the diagnosis of vitamin deficiency

Vitamin A	Plasma retinol
	Plasma carotene
Thiamin	RBC transketolase
	Urinary thiamin
Riboflavin	RBC glutathione reductase
	Urinary riboflavin
Pyridoxine	RBC glutamic oxaloacetic transaminase
	Urinary pyridoxic acid
Vitamin C	Leucocyte ascorbic acid
Vitamin D	Plasma 25 hydroxy cholecalciferol
Vitamin E	*In vitro* RBC haemolysis with H_2O_2
	Plasma tocopherol

Reproduced from Pennington C.R. (1988) *Therapeutic Nutrition*. Chapman & Hall Ltd, London.

Haematology

A haemoglobin estimation may indicate anaemia. Inspection of the blood film may prompt measurement of folate, vitamin B_{12} or iron.

Prolongation of the prothrombin time in the presence of normal liver function is indicative of vitamin K deficiency.

Immunology

Immunological parameters are also used to monitor malnourished patients who have reduced lymphocyte counts and loss of delayed hypersensitivity reactions on skin testing. Unfortunately the latter lacks specificity, anergy being a common feature in many diseases associated with malnutriton.

Diagnostic approach

The diagnostic approaches to obesity and to specific nutrient deficiencies, e.g. vitamin B_{12}, folate or iron, have been covered in previous chapters. The evaluation of specific micronutrient deficiencies, such as pellagra and scurvy, are beyond the scope of this chapter.

Table 12.5 summarizes the approach to the malnourished patient.

Table 12.5 Investigation of the patient with malnutrition

Identify the cause		
Factor	*Disease*	*Method*
Poor diet	Anorexia nervosa	Dietary assessment
	Altered taste, e.g. malignancy	
	Anorexia due to disease	
Malabsorption	Impaired digestion, e.g. pancreatitis	Screen for malabsorption
	Impaired absorption, e.g. coeliac disease	
	Bacterial colonization	
Increased requirements	Sepsis	Screen for infection *or* malignancy
	Burns	
Cachexia	Malignancy	
Measure the deficit and nutrient requirements		
Anthropometry		
Biochemistry		
Haematology		
Management plan		
Treat underlying disease		
Commence nutritional support		

Chapter 13
Communicable Diseases

Introduction

Infections are a common cause of ill health. For convenience they can be considered under the following arbitrary headings.

Childhood infections

These include illnesses such as measles, rubella, mumps, chickenpox and whooping cough. Investigation is rarely required as the diagnosis can be made on clinical grounds. Rubella is an important exception if there has been contact with non-immune pregnant patients when confirmation is required because of the risk of fetal deformity and the implications for therapeutic abortion. Furthermore, mumps may present in an atypical fashion with aseptic meningitis. Confirmation of the infection can be achieved by serology in these patients.

Organ-specific infections

Infections of the urinary tract, respiratory tract and gastrointestinal tract, as well as of the liver, skin and central nervous system have been covered in the respective sections of this book. The reader is referred to these chapters for guidance on their investigation.

Pyrexia of unknown origin (PUO)

This term is used to describe a recurrent or persistently raised temperature for which the cause is not immediately apparent. Three groups of conditions merit consideration. These are: infections, such as tuberculosis (do not overlook reactivation in the elderly) and endocarditis; immunogenic (collagen–vascular) disease, including systemic lupus erythematosus (SLE) vasculitis of various forms; and neoplastic disease like lymphoma or hypernephroma. Drug fever and artifactual temperature (when the patient tries to mislead medical attendants by warming the thermometer on the radiator!) must also be considered, where appropriate.

The investigation of patients with PUO will depend on the associated clinical features and history. The methods used to investigate infectious causes are summarized below.

Infections in travellers from abroad

Whereas patients who have returned from a holiday in an underdeveloped country must be screened for the common infections outlined above, there are particular infectious hazards which must be considered. Top of the list in terms of potential importance are malaria, gastrointestinal infections with *Salmonella*

211

or *Shigella* and amoebiasis. Brucellosis and schistosomiasis are sometimes imported along with more exotic diseases requiring advice from specialist centres.

Glandular fever syndrome

Classical infectious mononucleosis characterized by pharyngeal pseudomembrane and lymphadenopathy is caused by the Epstein–Barr virus. It has long been known that a similar illness is associated with cytomegaloviral infection and toxoplasmosis. The seroconversion syndrome of HIV infection is another recently recognized cause.

AIDS syndrome

This illness is characterized by immunosuppression, particularly with impaired helper T-cell function. It is caused by infection with the human immunodeficiency virus (HIV), of which two types are currently recognized. The patient is susceptible to infection with *Pneumocystis carinii*, cytomegalovirus, *Toxoplasma*, cryptococcus and various other infectious agents, all of which present in unusual and virulent forms.

Diagnostic approach

Pyrexia of unknown origin

Preliminary investigation includes a chest X-ray, urine microscopy and culture, blood cultures, liver function tests and blood count.

Inflammatory change on the chest film prompts a search for atypical pneumonia. Abnormality of the liver function tests leads to ultrasonic investigation of the liver (looking for abscesses or tumour) and gallbladder, and, if appropriate, a screen for hepatitis.

Where endocarditis is considered, an echocardiogram may define the presence of vegetations. An indium-labelled leucocyte scan can help to identify a deep-seated abscess. A liver biopsy may be needed to investigate the possibility of cryptogenic disseminated tuberculosis; the same information can be gleaned from the marrow aspirate.

Markers of immune disease including the antinuclear factor sometimes suggest SLE.

Imaging techniques may then be needed to search for solid tumours or lymphoma.

Pyrexia in the foreign traveller

The diagnostic approach will be influenced by information about the itinerary and the time-lapse since returning to the UK.

Simple investigations should be undertaken as previously outlined in the section on PUO. These include chest X-ray, blood count, liver function tests, blood and urine culture.

A search for malarial parasites in a thick blood film is an important initial investigation. The blood film may also show eosinophilia early in schistosomiasis, which may point to the need for urine examination and rectal biopsy. Stool culture and microscopy and serology for brucellosis are also important.

Glandular fever syndrome

The blood film shows glandular fever cells—atypical monocytes with foamy cytoplasm.

The Paul–Bunnell test is positive, except in children. When it is negative Epstein–Barr virus antibodies are useful. The IgM antibody is indicative of acute infection; because the infection is common most adults have detectable IgG antibodies.

When tests for the Epstein–Barr virus are negative, screen for cytomegalovirus and *Toxoplasma*.

AIDS

Patients who are suspected of HIV infection should be asked for permission to screen for the HIV virus antibody (remember that 6–12 weeks may elapse before seroconversion occurs).

When the AIDS syndrome seems likely, special techniques, including bronchoscopy, are needed to look for *Pneumocystis* infections. Routine investigations in the symptomatic patient include chest X-ray, blood and stool culture and stool microscopy.

Index